Latest Advances in Diagnosis and Treatment of Women-Associated Cancers

There has been tremendous progress in cancer diagnosis and treatment methodologies, and this book focuses on major cancers of the cervix, breast, endometrium and the associated female reproductive system. It focuses on specific diagnostic techniques and treatment strategies including computational tools, nanomedicine, and the use of machine learning, artificial intelligence, big data and other latest techniques, including the evolution of these treatments over the years. Oncologists, cancer scientists and professionals will find using the content on cutting-edge interventions by experts in their field, significantly improving earlier diagnosis and treatment options.

Key Features:

- Helps to improve quality of life after treatment, as the focus of healthcare is shifting from curative methods to primary prevention of diseases, screening methods, and early detection and treatment.
- Appeals to clinicians and residents interested in exploring cutting-edge technology for early diagnoses and treatment of women-associated cancers.
- Features a chapter on the clinician's perspective on advanced diagnostic and treatment methods.

T0353556

Latest Advances in Diagnosis and Treatment of Women-Associated Cancers

Edited by

Dr. Shazia Rashid, PhD
Centre for Medical Biotechnology, Amity Institute of
Biotechnology (AIB), Amity University Uttar Pradesh, India

Dr. Ankur Saxena, PhD
Amity Institute of Biotechnology (AIB),
Amity University Uttar Pradesh, India

Dr. Sabia Rashid, MRCP, FRCPath
Queen Elizabeth Hospital and
Kings College Hospital London, UK

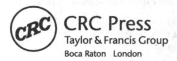

CRC Press
Taylor & Francis Group
Boca Raton   London

CRC Press is an imprint of the
Taylor & Francis Group, an **informa** business

First edition published 2023
by CRC Press
6000 Broken Sound Parkway NW, Suite 300, Boca Raton, FL 33487–2742

and by CRC Press
4 Park Square, Milton Park, Abingdon, Oxon, OX14 4RN

CRC Press is an imprint of Taylor & Francis Group, LLC

© 2023 selection and editorial matter, Shazia Rashid, Ankur Saxena and Sabia Rashid, individual chapters, the contributors

ISBN: 978-1-032-19636-7 (hbk)
ISBN: 978-1-032-19638-1 (pbk)
ISBN: 978-1-003-26017-2 (ebk)

DOI: 10.1201/9781003260172

Typeset in Times
by Apex CoVantage, LLC

For my family, who always stand by me, and the students who keep me inspired!

—Sh.R

For my family, who always comforts, consoles, and never complains; for their unwavering support!

—A.S

For my patients, who teach me humility and belief in humanity and keep me grounded!

—Sa.R

Contents

Preface

Women-associated cancers such as breast and cervical cancers are the top cancers affecting women worldwide. World Health Organization (WHO) in 2020 gave the mandate for elimination of cervical cancer as a public health problem and supporting governments in formulating comprehensive responses to the growing cancer burden. In order to address this global burden, early diagnosis is the best alternative for prevention. Currently, in most low- and middle-income countries (LMIC), cancer is diagnosed at an advanced stage, when treatment is generally less effective, more expensive and more disabling. The main triggers for women contacting health services are severity and persistence, which are also related to social sanctioning by people in women's networks.

Early diagnosis for symptomatic disease and screening of asymptomatic individuals can be important in managing gynaecological and breast cancers. Programs for early diagnosis consist of raising awareness about cancer symptoms, ensuring the capacity for rapid clinical and pathological diagnosis and timely referral to a site where effective treatment can be given.

Cancer management is generally more complex and conventional treatment can involve surgery, chemotherapy and radiotherapy. These treatments have their side effects and may not always be specific and targeted.

The past half century has seen tremendous progress in cancer diagnosis and treatment methodologies, mainly through advances in systemic therapy, and more recently using computational tools, nanotechnology, artificial intelligence (AI), machine learning (ML) and big data and other latest techniques.

This book is about cancers affecting women worldwide. It focuses on major cancers affecting women with special emphasis on breast and gynaecological cancers. It covers the advances in diagnosis and latest treatment and management strategies available for these cancers.

The book has been divided into chapters which focus on specific diagnostic and treatment strategies including new imaging techniques, computational tools, nanomedicine, use of ML, AI, big data and the evolution of these modalities over the years.

The target audiences for this book are oncologists, cancer scientists, academicians, public health researchers, physicians, PhD students and postgraduate students. This will serve as an easy-to-use resource in the area of cancer research, drug discovery, healthcare, public health, computational biology, ML, AI and nanotechnology for women-associated cancers. All the chapters have incorporated latest research and current methodologies to provide up-to-date information to the reader.

Acknowledgements

We would like to thank everyone who contributed to this project for their time and effort. We owe a debt of thanks to all of the authors for generously contributing their time and expertise, which has resulted in the successful completion of this book. We appreciate the reviewers' input in enhancing the chapters' quality, clarity and topic presentation. We are grateful to the team at CRC Taylor & Francis USA for their unwavering support. Last but not least, we are grateful for the continual support of our family and friends.

Shazia Rashid, PhD
Amity University Uttar Pradesh, Noida, India

Ankur Saxena, PhD
Amity University Uttar Pradesh, Noida, India

Sabia Rashid, MRCP, FRCPath
Queen Elizabeth Hospital and Kings College Hospital London, UK

About the Editors

Shazia Rashid is an academician, working as an assistant professor at the Amity Institute of Biotechnology (AIB) and adjunct faculty at the Amity Institute of Molecular Medicine and Stem Cells (AIMMSCR), Amity University Uttar Pradesh, Noida, India. She has ten years of experience as an academic in the areas of biomedical sciences and biotechnology. She obtained her PhD degree in biomedical sciences from the University of Ulster, UK. After completing her PhD, she worked as a post-doctoral fellow at the University of Ulster and later at the University of Oxford, UK. She has published more than 20 papers in international journals and published two books. She is an editorial board member and reviewer for several journals, like *Frontiers in Genetics Evolutionary and Population Genetics, Frontiers in Genetics,* section *Cancer Genetics and Oncogenomics, European Journal of Gynecological Oncology, Archives of Gynecology and Obstetrics,* and *Springer Nature*. Her areas of research interest include cancer biology and drug discovery, with an emphasis on human papillomavirus (HPV) infection and cervical cancer. Her research is focused on understanding the role of HPV in cervical cancer to identify novel methods for disease diagnosis and treatment.

Ankur Saxena is currently working as an assistant professor at Amity University Uttar Pradesh, Noida. He has 15 years of teaching experience at graduate and post-graduate levels and three years of industrial experience in the field of software development. He has published five books and more than 40 research articles in reputed journals. He is an editorial board member and reviewer for several journals. His research interests include cloud computing, big data, machine learning, evolutionary algorithms, software frameworks, design and analysis of algorithms and biometric identification.

Sabia Rashid is currently working as a consultant haematologist at Queen Elizabeth Hospital and Kings College Hospital in London, UK. She has over ten years of experience in treating haematological cancers, and her areas of expertise are acute leukaemia and myeloid disorders. She is actively involved in cancer research and is part of several clinical trials that are studying the biology and treatment of these cancers. She obtained her BSc and MBBS in India and then went on to work in the UK, where she obtained her post-graduate degree in haematology at Oxford University Hospitals. She is a member of the Royal College of Physicians and a Fellow of the Royal College of Pathologists, London. She is actively involved in teaching undergraduate and postgraduate medical students at Kings College University London, UK.

Contributors

Aditya Vikram Singh, Amity Institute of Biotechnology, Amity University, Noida, Uttar Pradesh, India

Ananya Bishnoi, Department of Allied Health Sciences, School of Health Sciences, University of Petroleum and Energy Studies (UPES), Energy Acres Building, Bidholi Dehradun, Uttarakhand, India

Ankur Saxena, Amity Institute of Biotechnology, Amity University, Noida, Uttar Pradesh, India

Anupama Avasthi, Amity Institute of Biotechnology, Amity University, Noida, Uttar Pradesh, India

Arushi Verma, Amity Institute of Biotechnology, Amity University, Noida, Uttar Pradesh, India

Ashfaq Ali Mir, University of Nice Sophia Antipolis, Nice, France

Ashish Mathur, Department of Physics, School of Engineering, University of Petroleum and Energy Studies (UPES), Energy Acres Building, Bidholi Dehradun, Uttarakhand, India

Asiya Khan, Centre for Medical Biotechnology, Amity Institute of Biotechnology, Amity University, Noida, Uttar Pradesh, India; Laboratory Oncology Unit, Rotary Cancer Centre, All India Institute of Medical Sciences, Ansari Nagar, New Delhi, India

Charu Sharma, Department of Obstetrics and Gynecology, All India Institute of Medical Sciences, Jodhpur, Rajasthan, India

Dhaval Kumar Srivastava, Amity Institute of Biotechnology, Amity University, Noida, Uttar Pradesh, India

Gunjan Vasant Bonde, Department of Pharmaceutical Sciences, School of Health Sciences, University of Petroleum and Energy Studies (UPES), Energy Acres Building, Bidholi Dehradun, Uttarakhand, India

Harsh Goel, Dr. B.R.A.-Institute Rotary Cancer Hospital, All India Institute of Medical Sciences, New Delhi, India

Jyoti Bala, Rapture Biotech International Pvt Ltd, Noida, Uttar Pradesh, India

Jyotirmoi Aich, School of Biotechnology and Bioinformatics, DY Patil Deemed to Be University, CBD Belapur, Navi Mumbai, Maharashtra, India

Malika Ranjan, Amity Institute of Molecular Medicine and Stem Cell Research (AIMMSCR), Amity University, Noida, India

Namyaa Kumar, Centre for Medical Biotechnology, Amity Institute of Biotechnology (AIB), Amity University Uttar Pradesh, India

Narrayan Raam Shankar, Dr. D.Y. Patil Biotechnology and Bioinformatics Institute, Dr. D.Y. Patil Vidyapeeth, Pune, Maharashtra, India

Navkiran Kaur, Amity Institute of Biotechnology, Amity University, Noida, Uttar Pradesh, India

Pawan K. Maurya, Department of Biochemistry, Central University of Haryana, Mahendergarh (Haryana), India

Pranay Tanwar, Dr. B.R.A.-Institute Rotary Cancer Hospital, All India Institute of Medical Sciences, New Delhi, India

Priyanka Mudaliar, School of Biotechnology and Bioinformatics, DY Patil Deemed to Be University, CBD Belapur, Navi Mumbai, Maharashtra, India

Rahul Kumar, Dr. B.R.A.-Institute Rotary Cancer Hospital, All India Institute of Medical Sciences, New Delhi, India

Rakesh Kumar, Dr. B.R.A.-Institute Rotary Cancer Hospital, All India Institute of Medical Sciences, New Delhi, India

Reetika Arora, Amity Institute of Biotechnology, Amity University Uttar Pradesh, Noida, India

Sabia Rashid, MRCP, FRCPath, Queen Elizabeth Hospital and Kings College Hospital London, UK

Safiya Arfi, Centre for Medical Biotechnology, Amity Institute of Biotechnology (AIB), Amity University Uttar Pradesh, India

Sandeep Sisodiya, Cellular and Molecular Diagnostics (Molecular Biology Group), ICMR-National Institute of Cancer Prevention and Research, Noida, India

Sangeeta Ballav, Cancer and Translational Research Laboratory, Dr. D.Y. Patil Biotechnology and Bioinformatics Institute, Dr. D.Y. Patil Vidyapeeth, Pune, Maharashtra, India

Shafina Siddiqui, School of Biotechnology and Bioinformatics, DY Patil Deemed to Be University, CBD Belapur, Navi Mumbai, Maharashtra, India

Shazia Rashid, Centre for Medical Biotechnology, Amity Institute of Biotechnology (AIB), Amity University Uttar Pradesh, India

Showket Hussain, ICMR-National Institute of Cancer Prevention and Research, Indian Council of Medical Research Department of Health Research, Ministry of Health and Family Welfare, Govt of India, Noida, India

Smriti Arora, Department of Allied Health Sciences, School of Health Sciences, University of Petroleum and Energy Studies (UPES), Energy Acres Building, Bidholi Dehradun, Uttarakhand, India

Somorjit Singh Ningombam, Dr. B.R.A.-Institute Rotary Cancer Hospital, All India Institute of Medical Sciences, New Delhi, India

Sonam Tulsyan, Cellular and Molecular Diagnostics (Molecular Biology Group), ICMR-National Institute of Cancer Prevention and Research, Noida, India

Soumya Basu, Cancer and Translational Research Laboratory, Dr. D.Y. Patil Biotechnology and Bioinformatics Institute, Dr. D.Y. Patil, Vidyapeeth, Pune, Maharashtra, India

Umme Abiha, Department of Obstetrics and Gynecology, All India Institute of Medical Sciences, Jodhpur, Rajasthan, India

Vishakha Kasherwal, Cellular and Molecular Diagnostics (Molecular Biology Group), ICMR-National Institute of Cancer Prevention and Research, Noida, India; Amity Institute of Molecular Medicine and Stem Cell Research, Amity University, Noida, India

Abbreviations

CHAPTER 01

5-FU-5	Fluorouracil
ADP	Adenosine diphosphate
ATM	Ataxia-telangiectasia (A-T) mutated
BAX	Bcl-2–associated X-protein
BRCA	Breast cancer gene
BRIP1	BRCA1 interacting protein 1
CA125	Cancer antigen 125
CRP	Complement regulatory protein
CT	Computerized tomography
DBT	Digital breast tomosynthesis
DNA	Deoxyribonucleic acid
EGFR	Epidermal growth factor receptor
EOC	Epithelial ovarian cancer
ER	Estrogen
FDA	US Food and Drug Administration
FIGO	International Federation of Gynaecology and Obstetrics
FRα	Folate receptor
HE4	Human epididymis protein 4
HER2	Human epidermal growth factor
HIC	High-income countries
HPV	Human papillomavirus
IMRT	Intensity-modulated radiation therapy
LEEP	Loop electrosurgical excision procedure
LMICs	Low- and middle-income countries
MRI	Magnetic resonance imaging
mTOR	Mammalian target of rapamycin
PAP	Papanicolaou test
PARP	Poly-adenosine diphosphate-ribose polymerase
PCOS	Polycystic ovary syndrome
PD-1	Programmed cell death 1

PET	Positron emission tomography
PI3K	Phosphoinositide 3-kinase
PR	Progesterone
RNA	Ribose nucleic acid
SERD	Selective estrogen receptor downregulator
TVUS	Transvaginal ultrasound
VEGF	Vascular endothelial growth factor
WHO	World Health Organization

CHAPTER 02

BRCA	Breast cancer gene
CUR	Curcumin
DES	Diethylstilbestrol
FDA	US Food and Drug Administration
GLOBOCAN	Global Cancer Observatory
HPV	Human papillomavirus
MAP kinase	Mitogen-activated protein kinase
MOF	Metal organic framework
NP	Nanoparticle
PET	Positron emission tomography
PLA	Polylactic acid
PLGA	Poly-(lactic-co-glycolic acid)
QC	Quercitin
WHO	World Health Organization

CHAPTER 03

2D	Two-dimensional
3D	Three-dimensional
ABUS	Automated breast ultrasound
AJCC	American Joint Committee on Cancer
AVBS	Automated breast volume scanner
BIRADS	Breast Imaging Reporting and Data System
CEDM	Contrast-enhanced digital mammography
CEUS	Contrast-enhanced ultrasound

CT	Computer tomography
CTLM	Computed tomography laser mammography
DBT	Digital breast tomosynthesis
DWI	Diffusion-weighted imaging
FDA	US Food and Drug Administration
FDG	Fluorodeoxyglucose
IDSI	Imaging Diagnostic Systems, Inc.
MRE	Magnetic resonance elastography
MRI	Magnetic resonance imaging
MRS	Magnetic resonance spectroscopy
NCCN	National Comprehensive Cancer Network
NIR	Near-infrared range
PEM	Positron emission mammography
PET	Positron emission tomography
SPECT	Single-photon emission computed tomography
US	Ultrasound

CHAPTER 04

ADCC	Antibody-dependent cell-mediated cytotoxicity
APCs	Antigen-presenting cells
BRCA	Breast cancer gene
CTL A-4	Cytotoxic T lymphocyte antigen-4
DCs	Dendritic cells
DSBs	Double strand breaks
ER	Estrogen receptor
FDA	US Food and Drug Administration
HER2	Human epidermal growth factor receptor 2
ICI	Immune checkpoint inhibitors
LAG3	Lymphocyte activation gene 3
NK cell	Natural killer cell
NKT cell	Natural killer T cell
OR	Objective response
ORR	Overall response rate
PARPi	Poly-(ADP-ribose) polymerase inhibitor
PD-L1	Programmed death-ligand 1
PD1	Programmed cell death 1
PFS	Progression free survival
TCR	T-cell antigen receptor

| **TNBC** | Triple negative breast cancer |
| **Tregs** | Regulatory T cell |

CHAPTER 05

3D	3-dimensional
3D QSAR	3D quantitative structure-activity relationship
ADMET	Absorption, distribution, metabolism, excretion and toxicity
BC	Breast cancer
c-MET	Mesenchymal epithelial transition
CADD	Computer-aided drug designing
CoMFA	Comparative molecular field analysis
CoMSIA	Comparative molecular similarity index
CYP	Activity of cytochrome
H	Hydrogen
HDACs	Histone deacetylase
HER2	Human epidermal growth factor receptor 2
HIV	Human immunodeficiency virus
HPV	Human papillomavirus
LBDD	Ligand-based drug designing
MAPK	Mitogen activated protein kinase
MD	Molecular dynamics
NMR	Nuclear magnetic resonance
PDB	Protein data bank
PI3K	Phosphoinositide-3 kinase
PPI	Protein-protein interaction
Rb	Retinoblastoma
RO5	Rule of five
SBDD	Structure-based drug designing
TGF-β	Transforming growth factor-β
VEGF	Vascular endothelial growth factor
VS	Virtual screening

CHAPTER 06

| **ADC** | Antibody-drug conjugate |
| **BC** | Breast cancer |

CC	Cervical cancer
CG	Chorionic gonadotropin
DNA	Deoxyribonucleic acid
DOX	Doxorubicin
EGFR	Epidermal growth factor receptor
EPR	Enhanced permeability and retention
HER	Human epidermal growth factor receptor
LHRH	Luteinizing hormone–releasing hormone
MAPK	Mitogen-activated protein kinase
MRI	Magnetic resonance imaging
NPs	Nanoparticles
OC	Ovarian cancer
PAI-1	Plasminogen activator inhibitor-1
PCL-PLA-TPGS	Polycaprolactone-polylactic acid-d-α-tocopheryl polyethylene glycol 1000 succinate
PDCs	Peptide-drug conjugates
PET	Photon emission computed tomography
PI3K/AKT	Phosphatidylinositol 3-kinases/protein kinase B
PLNs	Polymer-coated lipid nanoparticles
QDs	Quantum dots
SPECT	Single photon emission computed tomography
SPIONs	Superparamagnetic iron oxide nanoparticles
US	United States
VEGFR	Vascular endothelial growth factor receptor

CHAPTER 07

AR-V7	Androgen receptor splice variant 7 gene
BRAF	Human gene that encodes a protein called B-Raf
BRAF	Encodes a protein belonging to the RAF family of serine/threonine protein kinases
BRCA1	Breast cancer type 1 susceptibility protein
c-MET	Tyrosine-protein kinase Met
CKIT	Proto-oncogene c-KIT, the gene encoding the receptor tyrosine kinase protein known as tyrosine-protein kinase KIT
DNA	Deoxyribonucleic acid
EGFR	Estimated glomerular filtration rate
ESCAT	ESMO Scale for Clinical Actionability of Molecular Targets

ESMO	European Society for Medical Oncology
ESTs	Expressed sequence tags
EWAS	Epigenome-wide association study
FFPE	Preservation and preparation for biopsy specimens
GENCODE	Database for Genes and Genomes
GRAIL	American biotechnology and pharmaceutical company
GTEx	Genotype-tissue expression datasets
H3K27ac	Marker for active enhancers and a great indicator of enhancer activity
HGF	Tyrosine-protein kinase Met or hepatocyte growth factor receptor, a protein that in humans is encoded by the MET gene
HISAT	Read alignment program for mapping RNA-Seq data
HRD	Homologous recombination deficiency
LINE-1	Long interspersed nuclear element-1
MCF7	Epithelial cancer cell line derived from breast adenocarcinoma
PDL-1	Programmed death-ligand 1 (PD-L1) is a 40kDa type 1 transmembrane protein
PGAP2	Post-GPI attachment to proteins 2, a protein coding gene
PIK3CA	Phosphatidylinositol-4,5-bisphosphate 3-kinase catalytic subunit alpha
PIQRAY	Cancer medicine used to treat postmenopausal women and men with breast cancer
RNA	Ribonucleic acid
RUBRACA	PARP inhibitor used as an anti-cancer agent
STAR	Read alignment program for mapping RNA-Seq data
TNBC	Triple-negative breast cancer
TPD52	Tumour protein D52, a protein coding gene
TWAS	Transcriptome-wide association study
UCSC	University of California, Santa Cruz

CHAPTER 08

CADD	Computer-aided drug designing
E6-AP	E6-associated protein
GVHD	Graft versus host disease
HPV	Human papillomavirus
KEGG	Kyoto Encyclopedia of Genes and Genomes

NCBI	National Center for Biotechnology Information
NMR	spectroscopy nuclear magnetic resonance spectroscopy
pI	Isoelectric point
SOPMA	Self-optimized method with alignment
TP 53	Tumour protein 53

CHAPTER 09

AI	Artificial Intelligence
ANN	Artificial neural network
BF	Best First trees
BOT	Benign ovarian tumour
CA125	Cancer antigen 125
CEA	Carcinoembryonic Antigen
CNN	Convolutional neural network
CT	Computed Tomography
DCE	Dynamic contrast-enhanced
DCE- MR	Dynamic contrast-enhanced- magnetic resonance
DD-ResNet	Deep dilated residual network
DDCNN	Deep dilated convolutional neural network
DDNN	Deep deconvolutional neural network
DM	DNA methylation
DMI	Deep myometrial invasion
DMIMS	Diagnosis model and information monitoring system
DSC	Dice similarity coefficient
DTBDS	Decision tree based on decision support degree
EC	Endometrial cancer
EOC	Epithelial ovarian cancer
GE	Gene expression
GP	General Practitioner
HE4	Human epididymis protein 4
HPV	Human Papillomavirus
ID- 3	Iterative Dichotomiser 3
K- SVM	Kernel-based Support vector machines
KNN	K-Nearest Neighbour
LBK	Lazy k-nearest neighbour
LDA	Linear discriminant analysis
LNI	Lymph node involvement
MALDI	Matrix-Assisted Laser Desorption/Ionization

ML	Machine Learning
MRI	Magnetic resonance imaging
MRMR	Minimum redundancy–maximum relevance
NCCN	National Comprehensive Cancer Network
OC	Ovarian cancer
PaLNI	Para-aortic Lymph node involvement
PGSO	Particle genetic swarm optimization
SMO	Sequential minimal optimization
SVM	Support vector machines
SVM- lin	Support vector machines with linear kernel
SVM- rbf	Support vector machines with radial basis function kernel
T1W	T1-weighted
T2W	T2-weighted
UCI	UC Irvine Machine Learning
WDBC	Wisconsin Diagnosis Breast Cancer
XG- Boost	Extreme Gradient Boost

CHAPTER 10

ADA	Adenosine deaminase
AI	Artificial intelligence
CIN	Cervical intraepithelial neoplasia
CKC	Cold knife conization
CT	Computed tomography
EVs	Extracellular vesicles
HPV	Human papillomavirus
LBC	Liquid-based cytology
LEEP	Loop electrosurgical excision procedure
ML	Machine learning
MRI	Magnetic resonance imaging
PEDF	Pigment epithelium-derived factor
PET	Positron emission tomography
RF	Radio frequency
SCID	Severe combined immunodeficiency
SPIONs	Superparamagnetic iron oxide
T-zone	Transition zone
TKIs	Tyrosine kinase inhibitors
VIA	Visual inspection with acetic acid
VILI	Visual inspection with Lugol's iodine
WSI	Whole-slide imaging

Glossary

Antiangiogenic agents Can be used to effectively regulate the tumour vasculature and reduce vascular growth for a certain amount of time.

Antineoplastic agents Drugs that are used to inhibit the development of tumours.

Apoptosis Programmed cell death in a multicellular organism to eliminate redundant or abnormal cells from the body.

BF Tree method Friedman, Hastie and Tibshirani introduced a relatively innovative and robust tree-based learning method in the year 2000, which was refined by Haijian in 2007. A root node, internal nodes, and leaves make up the structure of the BF Tree. The basic divide-and-conquer approach is used to grow the trees in the BF Tree algorithm.

Binding pocket A cavity of a protein which aids in binding of ligands.

Bispecific antibodies A type of artificial antibody that binds to two distinct antigens at the same time.

Brachytherapy Uses radioactive sources to destroy cancer cells and shrink tumours.

Breast imaging A sub-speciality of diagnostic radiology that involves imaging of the breasts for screening or diagnostic purposes. There are various methods of breast imaging using a variety of technologies.

CADD An in silico approach for drug designing.

Cardiomyopathy An acquired or hereditary disease of the heart muscle.

CART cell therapy Treatment in which a patient's T cells (a type of immune system cell) are genetically modified to attack cancer cells.

CDx test Companion diagnostics test.

Chemotherapy A type of treatment of cancer that involves the administration of one or a combination of two or more cytotoxic drugs that has the ability to destroy or inhibit the growth of cancer cells, thereby reducing tumour growth.

ChIP-Seq Chromatin immunoprecipitation with massively parallel DNA sequencing to identify the binding sites of DNA-associated proteins.

Colposcopy A procedure to closely examine the cervix, vulva and vagina for the presence of a disease; usually performed with the help of a device called colposcope.

Computed tomography (CT) Also called computerized tomography or computerized axial tomography (CAT); an imaging procedure which utilizes special x-ray equipment for creating detailed pictures, or scans, of areas inside the body.

Conization   A surgery that involves removing a cone-shaped portion of aberrant tissue from the cervix.

Conventional   Behaving in a traditional or normal way.

Convolutional neural network (CNN)   A type of artificial neural network used in image recognition and processing that is specifically designed to process pixel data.

Cryoablation   A process that involves freezing and destroying aberrant cells or sick tissue with extremely cold gas.

Crystallography   A branch of science that deals with characterization of crystal.

Curettage   The use of a curette, especially on the lining of the uterus.

Cystoscopy   A procedure to examine lining of bladder and urethra.

Cytoreduction   A type of cancer treatment that tries to lower the amount of cancer cells by removing the main tumour or metastatic deposits to lessen the tumour's immunosuppressive load, relieve symptoms and avoid complications.

Deep deconvolutional neural network (DDNN)   An encoder and a decoder are two crucial components of an end-to-end architecture.

Deep dilated convolutional neural network (DDCNN)   A technique that expands the kernel (input) by inserting holes between its consecutive elements.

Dice similarity coefficient (DSC)   The quotient of similarity which ranges between 0 and 1 and can be viewed as a similarity measure over sets.

Digital breast tomosynthesis   A type of mammography that creates three-dimensional images of the breasts using a low-dose x-ray equipment and computer reconstructions.

DNA methylation   A process by which methyl groups are added to the DNA molecule.

Docking   A process used to predict the interaction between protein and ligand; a method to predict preferred orientation (bond formation) of subjected molecules.

Drug discovery   The process of identification of potential new medicines are identified using wide range of scientific disciplines, including biology, chemistry and pharmacology.

Dynamic contrast enhanced (DCE) CT   Following an intravenous bolus of iodinated contrast medium (300 mg/mL) administered at 2 mL/sec, the DCE-CT approach involves the acquisition of a dynamic sequence of brief spiral acquisitions centred on the SPN with the patient breath-holding.

Dysplasia   Abnormal growth and proliferation of cells within a tissue or organ.

Elucidate   To make something clearer by explaining it.

Endometriosis   A condition in which the tissue that borders the uterus develops outside of it.

Epigenetics   The study of the changes in the gene activity without involving alterations in the DNA sequence.

Erythema   Skin redness.

FDA approved   Approved by the US Food and Drug Administration.

Gene expression   The process of information transfer from a gene into a functional gene product (protein or non-coding RNA), enabling the ultimate effect on the phenotype.

Genealogy of disease   Family history consisting of information about disorders from which direct blood relatives of the patient have suffered.

Genomics   An interdisciplinary branch of biology that concerned with the large-scale study of the genome of an organism.

Gynaecological cancers   Cancer of the reproductive organs of a women.

Herbal informatics   Informatics-based approach for proposing herbal drugs.

Homology modelling   A process used to construct tertiary structure of protein based upon the sequence homologs of available structure of protein or template.

Hybrid particle genetic swarm optimization (PGSO)   A computational strategy for solving problems by iteratively trying to enhance a potential solution in terms of a quality metric.

Hyperplasia   Enlargement of an organ or tissue due to an increase in the rate of cell proliferation.

Hysterectomy   Surgical removal of the uterus. The cervix, ovaries, fallopian tubes and other surrounding structures may also be removed.

IBK method   Instead of building a model, the instance based learner algorithm makes a forecast for a test case just in time.

Imaging modalities   Medical imaging techniques that utilize a certain physical mechanism to detect patient internal signals that reflect either anatomical structures or physiological events.

Immune checkpoint inhibitors   A type of drug that blocks checkpoint proteins, resulting in its binding with partner proteins.

Immunotherapeutics   A type of drugs which helps your immune system to fight with disease.

Immunotherapy   A type of cancer therapy related with immune suppression/activation.

Intensity-modulated RT (IMRT)   Linear accelerators are used in this therapy to safely deliver precise radiation to a tumour while limiting the exposure to surrounding normal tissue.

Intrathecal chemotherapy   Anticancer medications are injected into the fluid-filled area between the thin tissue layers that surround the brain and spinal cord during this chemotherapy.

K-means clustering   A type of unsupervised learning, which is used when you have unlabelled data (i.e., data without defined categories or groups).

KNN   "K-nearest neighbor," a supervised machine learning algorithm used to solve both classification and regression problem statements.

Laparoscopy   A surgical operation in which a fibre-optic tool is introduced through the abdominal wall to allow small-scale surgery or to see the organs in the abdomen.

Laser ablation   The technique of eliminating cells from a solid (or occasionally liquid) tumour/cell mass by irradiating it with a laser beam.

Ligands/hits   Potential drug (an in silico term), yet in testing phase.

Linear discriminant analysis (LDA)   An algorithm primarily used to minimize the number of features before classification to a more manageable quantity.

Logistic regression   A sort of statistical analysis (also known as a logit model) commonly used for predictive analytics and modelling, as well as machine learning applications.

Loop electrosurgical excision procedure (LEEP)   This procedure removes cells and tissue from a woman's lower vaginal tract using a wire loop heated by electric current.

Lymphadenectomy   Swelling of lymph nodes.

Machine learning   A branch of artificial intelligence focusing on the use of data and algorithms to imitate the way that humans learn, gradually improve its accuracy.

Magnetic resonance imaging (MRI)   A non-invasive imaging technique that uses magnetic field and radio waves to create comprehensive three-dimensional images of anatomy of body

Malignancy   The state or presence of a malignant tumour, or cancer.

Malignant   A condition in which tumour cells spread to the other parts of body distinct from the source of origin.

Mammogram   A diagnostic and screening procedure that involves the use of low-energy x-rays to scan the human breast.

Mammography   A technique using x-rays to diagnose and locate tumours of the breasts.

Mass spectrometry   An analytic tool used to identify chemical substances based on their mass to charge ratio.

Mastectomy   The medical or surgical procedure employed for partial or complete removal of one or both breasts as a part of surgical treatment of breast cancer.

Metastasis   Spread of cancer cells from the site of primary tumour to other organs or tissues of the body.

Metastasize (of a cancer)   The spread to other sites in the body by metastasis.

Microarray   A technique used to detect the expression of a set of genes at once.

MicroRNA   A single-stranded non-coding RNA molecule that regulates RNA silencing and post-transcriptional control gene expression.

Microwave imaging   An imaging technique using nonionizing electromagnetic (EM) signals in the frequency range of hundreds of megahertz to a few gigahertz.

Minimum redundancy maximum relevance (MRMR)   A feature selection method that favours features that have a strong correlation with the class (output) but a low correlation with one another.

Molecular dynamics simulation   A computational approach to calculate the physical movement of atoms present in the protein molecule in their native environment.

Monoclonal antibody   Binds to only one substance.

Morbidity   The condition of suffering from a disease or medical condition.

Mortality   The number of deaths in one period of time or in one place.

Multifactorial   Involving or dependent on a number of factors, especially genetic or environmental factors.

Multiparametric MRI   A method of merging T2-weighted (T2WI), diffusion weighted (DWI), dynamic contrast enhanced (DCEI), and, if needed, MR spectroscopy (MRSI) images to try to generate an ideal three-dimensional (3D) prostate image.

Mutagens   Chemical chemicals or kinds of radiation (such as ultraviolet light or x-rays) that produce irreversible and heritable changes (mutations) in the genetic material of cells, deoxyribonucleic acid (DNA).

Naïve Bayes ML algorithm   A supervised learning algorithm for addressing classification issues; it is based on the Bayes theorem and is mostly utilized in text classification tasks that require a large training dataset.

Nanocarriers   These are drug-loaded carriers having particle size in colloidal (typically <500 nm).

Nanomedicine, or nano drug delivery systems   A material in the nanoscale range that is employed to load and then deliver the drug in the body after administration. The loaded drug can be a diagnostic agent or any drug that is used for treatment of disease.

Neuropathy   Weakness, numbness and pain from nerve damage, usually in the hands and feet.

NGS technologies   Next generation sequencing technologies to determine order or targeted genome or transcriptome.

Nipple-sparing mastectomy   The nipple, areola, and breast skin are all preserved after a nipple-sparing mastectomy.

Novel   New and different.

Oncogene   Mutated, cancer-causing form of a normal gene.

Oncoprotein   A protein encoded by viral oncogene.

Optical imaging   Uses light and special properties of photons to obtain detailed images of organs, tissues, cells and even molecules.

Pap smear   A procedure in which a small brush is used to gently remove cells from the surface of the cervix and the area around it so they can be checked under a microscope for cervical cancer or cell changes that may lead to cervical cancer.

Peritoneal metastasis   Cancer that has migrated to the peritoneum from other organs. It appears as soft-tissue lumps that are nodular or plaque-like in appearance.

PET scan (positron emission tomography)   Evaluates organ and tissue functions by using small amounts of radioactive chemicals called radiotracers or radiopharmaceuticals to detect the early development of disease.

Pharmacokinetics   Branch of pharmacology concerned with the activity of foreign chemicals within the body from absorption to till excretion.

Pharmacological activity   Study which describes the effect of a drug on the living bodies.

Pharmacophore modelling   A process used in virtual screening of compounds based on steric and electronic features of the ligand.

Polyps   Tissue growths that resemble little, flat bumps or miniature mushroom-like stems. They generally develop in the lining of the colon.

Prevalence   The fact or condition of being prevalent; commonness.

Proteomics   An interdisciplinary branch of biology that concerned with the extensive study of proteins of an organism.

Radial basis function kernel   A popular function used in various kernelized learning algorithms; particularly used in support vector machine classification.

Radical trachelectomy   Surgery to remove the cervix, nearby tissue and lymph nodes, and the upper part of the vagina.

Radiology   The medical discipline that uses medical imaging to diagnose and treat diseases within the bodies of animals and humans.

Radiotherapy   A technique used in treatment of disease, especially cancer, using x-rays or similar forms of radiation.

Random forest   Also known as random decision forests; an ensemble learning method for classification, regression, and other problems that works by training a large number of decision trees.

Reinforcement learning (RL)   An area of ML concerned with how intelligent agents ought to take actions in an environment in order to maximize the notion of cumulative reward.

RNA-Seq   Sequencing technique to quantify ribonucleic acid.

Saline infusion sonohysterography Involves injecting a tiny quantity of saline (salt solution) into the uterus (or womb) to allow the endometrium (uterine lining) to be seen clearly on an ultrasound scan.

Salpingo-oophorectomy Surgical removal of the ovaries and fallopian tubes.

Sequential minimal optimization (SMO) is an algorithm for solving the quadratic programming (QP) problem that arises during the training of support-vector machines (SVM).

Skin-sparing mastectomy The breast tissue is removed while most of the healthy breast skin is left in a skin-sparing mastectomy.

Sonography A procedure that uses high-energy sound waves to look at tissues and organs inside the body.

Supervised learning A type of machine learning in which machines are trained using well "labelled" training data and on the basis of this data it predicts the output.

Support vector machine (SVM) A supervised machine learning algorithm used for both classification and regression.

Support vector machines with linear (SVM-lin) Used for linearly separable data, which means if a dataset can be classified into two classes by using a single straight line, then such data is termed as linearly separable data, and classifier is used called a linear SVM classifier.

Synergistic Related to incorporation of two or more agents.

Target deconvolution A retrospective approach based on phenotype of disease used to identify a molecular target.

Target validation A process involving various techniques which aim to demonstrate the effect of a drug on its target and its therapeutic benefits.

Theranostics A combination of therapeutics and diagnostics; describes the simultaneous administration of at least two drugs, one of which is used for diagnosis of cancer and another administered for the treatment of cancer/metastatic tumours.

Tomosynthesis An imaging, or x-ray, technique that can be used to screen for early signs of breast cancer in people with no symptoms.

Transcriptomics It is technique used to study the complete set of mRNA of an organism.

Transvaginal ultrasound (TVUS) Internal scan of female reproductive tract. A small ultrasonic probe, known as a transducer, is inserted into the vaginal canal to create detailed images of the pelvic organs.

Tumour An abnormal mass of tissue that forms when cells grow and divide more than they should or do not die when they should.

Ulceration Formation of a break on the skin or on surface of organ.

Unsupervised learning   The use of artificial intelligence (AI) algorithms to identify patterns in data sets containing data points that are neither classified nor labelled.

Vaccine   A biological preparation that provides active acquired immunity to a particular infectious disease.

WDBC   Wisconsin Breast Cancer Database for Diagnosis; a digitized image of a fine needle aspirate (FNA) of a breast mass used to compute features which define the image's cell nuclei.

Weka software   A set of machine learning methods for data mining tasks that includes tools for data preparation, classification, regression, clustering, association rules mining and visualization. It is an open-source software released under the GNU General Public License.

Women-specific cancer   The collective term used to describe cancers of body organs that are specific to female/women anatomy.

XG-Boost   Xtreme Gradient Boosting; a decision-tree-based ensemble machine learning algorithm that uses a gradient boosting framework whilst providing a parallel tree boosting (also known as GBDT, GBM).

Overview of Traditional Methods of Diagnosis and Treatment for Women-Associated Cancers

1

Malika Ranjan, Namyaa Kumar, Safiya Arfi and Shazia Rashid

Contents

DOI: 10.1201/9781003260172-1

INTRODUCTION

Cancer is a one of the leading cause of mortality worldwide especially among women in both low- and middle-income countries (LMICs) and high-income countries which has been attributed to the increasing exposure to associated risk factors like diet and lifestyle changes, alcohol consumption, smoking tobacco, exposure to industrial chemicals, changes in reproductive patterns, like older age at first pregnancy and fewer or no childbirths [1]. Among different women-associated cancers, breast cancer has the highest incidence and death rate, followed by gynaecological cancers (cervical, endometrial, and ovarian cancers) [2]. Cancer is a multifactorial disease where genetic susceptibility, environment, nutrition, and lifestyle risk factors interact and contribute to its occurrence. At the molecular level, cancer is driven by genetic and epigenetic alterations that cause cells to over proliferate, invade the surrounding tissues and metastasize.

In the past, most cancers were treated with surgery, radiation, and chemotherapy, however, with the passage of time and advances in diagnosis and treatment modalities, combination of treatments was observed to be more effective. Currently, precision cancer treatment (targeted therapy) and immune-mediated therapies including cancer vaccines, engineered immune cells, and checkpoint inhibitors and gene therapy have been introduced for the treatment of different women-associated cancers [3–5]. Similarly, hormonal therapies are helpful in treating hormone receptors positive cancer such as breast cancer by limiting hormonal growth factors [6]. Also, recent advances in genetic engineering and stem cell research have created the foundation for genetically engineering stem cells with anti-tumour effects as therapeutic vehicles besides dendritic cell-based immunotherapy [4,7].

In addition, since most women-associated cancers including breast cancer, cervical, ovarian and uterine, are diagnosed at a later stage, prevention and early detection interventions including those to eliminate or reduce cancer risk factors or increase access to affordable, good quality diagnostic and treatment services are needed in all countries especially in LMICs with weak and under-resourced health systems.

In this chapter, we summarize the present status, burden and trends of different women-associated cancers worldwide. The chapter also highlights traditional methods and some latest advances in the diagnosis and treatment of women-associated cancers.

CANCER PREVALENCE

Among women, cancer is the second leading cause of death worldwide and in the United States, Europe and the western Pacific region [1]. More than 2 million women are diagnosed with breast cancer and genital tract cancer each year worldwide. There were approximately 9.2 million new cancer cases and 4.4 million deaths among females worldwide in 2020, with breast cancer ranking first for incidence and for mortality in the vast majority of countries, followed by cervical cancer, uterine cancers and ovarian cancer [2].

Besides breast cancer, gynaecological cancers like cervical cancer, endometrial cancer, ovarian cancer and vaginal and vulvar cancer are important contributors to women cancer mortality. Cervical cancer is the fourth most common cancer among women worldwide [8]. It is also the fourth most common cause of cancer death worldwide, with 90% of the global cancer burden being borne by LMICs [2]. The global burden and trend in incidence and mortality of different women-associated cancer is rising fast and varies greatly with geographic location [9–13] (Figure 1.1A, 1.1B). The burden of cancer among women could be substantially reduced in both HICs and LMICs through implementation of effective screening and prevention strategies, including tobacco control, vaccination and improved access to quality treatment.

WOMEN-ASSOCIATED CANCERS

The two main types of women-associated cancers include breast cancer and gynaecologic cancer, which affects reproductive organs of the women. Gynaecologic cancer includes cervical, ovarian, uterine, and vaginal and vulvar cancers.

Breast cancer is the type of cancer originating from the cell lining of the milk-forming ducts of the breast (ductal carcinoma) or from lobules in the glandular tissue of the breast (lobular carcinoma). Breast cancer has several subtypes based on the expression level of the receptors such as progesterone, estrogen and HER-2/neu (human epidermal growth factor receptor), and are classified into three groups [14]:

- Hormone receptor (estrogen and progesterone) sensitive (ER+ or PR+).
- Human epidermal growth factor–sensitive (HER2+).
- Triple-negative breast cancer (ER–, PR–, HER2–).

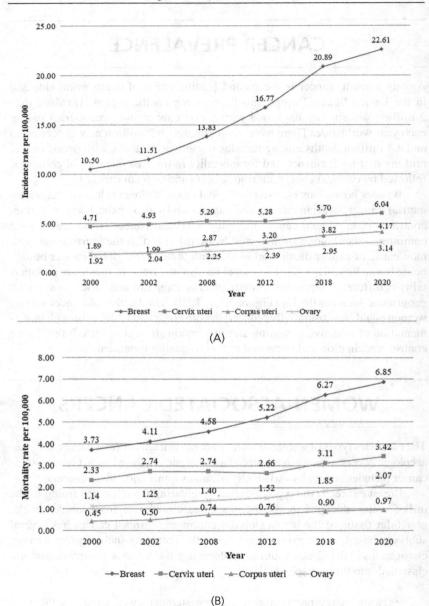

FIGURE 1.1   Global trend in incidence (A) and mortality (B) for different women-associated cancers from 2000 to 2020.

The main factors that influence the risk for breast cancer in women include old age, genetic mutations, reproductive history, personal history of breast/ovarian cancer or any non-cancerous breast diseases, previous treatment involving radiation therapy and other lifestyle factors (diet, weight, alcohol consumption). Thus, regular screening mammography at the age of 40 and above might reduce the risk of breast cancer mortality in average-risk women.

Cervical cancer is cancer arising from the cervix, a part of the uterus in female reproductive organ. The persistent infection of the human papillomavirus (high-risk subtypes of HPV, HPV-16 and HPV-18) is the principal cause of almost all cervical cancers whereas risk factors such as early marriage, promiscuity, bad genital hygiene and so forth are other well-known causes [15]. Cervical cancer, though highly prevalent cancer, can be prevented primarily by avoiding HPV infection through HPV vaccination and undergoing screening programs. The commonly used bivalent (Cervarix), quadrivalent (Gardasil) and 9-valent HPV vaccine (Gardasil-9) have shown greater (90%) efficacy in protecting against infection of HPV-16 and HPV-18, which are associated with high-grade cervical dysplasia. The implementation of formal screening programs in developed countries has helped reduce incidents and mortality of cervical cancer to nearly half in the past 30 years [15].

Ovarian cancer refers to any cancerous growth that originates in the ovaries, or in related areas of the fallopian tube and the peritoneum. The cause of ovarian cancer is multifactorial which mainly include genetic, immunologic, and environmental factors. Some most common causes of ovarian cancer are inherited gene changes (including BRCA1, BRCA2, BRIP1, RAD51C, RAD51D and genes associated with Lynch syndrome), postmenopausal hormone replacement therapy and endometriosis [16]. The use of oral contraceptives, like birth control pills, has been shown to dramatically reduce the risk of ovarian cancer and endometrial cancer [17].

Endometrial cancer is cancer that arises in the layer of cells that form the lining (endometrium) of the uterus. Most uterine cancers are endometrial cancers and the women of all ages (especially with PCOS) are at risk of endometrial cancer, however, its incidence is high after menopause. Risk factors include family history, diabetes mellitus, endometrial hyperplasia (have a 1%–3% chance of progressing to endometrial cancer) and Lynch syndrome among many others [16].

Vulvar cancer is usually formed as a lump or ulcer in the vagina that often causes itching. Cancer of the fallopian tubes is a rare gynaecological cancer, which starts in the fallopian tubes and generally affects women between the ages of 50 and 60.

DIAGNOSIS AND TREATMENT OF WOMEN-ASSOCIATED CANCERS

The diagnosis and treatment of different women-associated cancers depends primarily on factors like size of tumour, stage and type of cancer, age and overall health of the patient and on locally available resources required for its treatment. Different types of imaging tests such as x-ray, computerized tomography (CT), magnetic resonance imaging (MRI) and positron emission tomography (PET-CT) scans, mammography are routinely used to detect cancer in the early stage, determine the extent of its spread and check if the treatment is working. However, the diagnosis and prognosis also depend on the type of cancer. Figure 1.2 depicts tools and techniques that are used for diagnosis of different women-associated cancers.

TREATMENT MODALITIES

The selection of treatment of different women-associated cancers, and their progress depends largely on cancer type, locality, and stage of progression. Some of the most traditional and widely used treatment for cancer involves surgery, radiation and chemotherapy or a combination of therapies. Figure 1.3 depicts the traditional treatment for specific cancers affecting women.

Surgery

Surgery is one of the most common and conventional treatments of many benign and malignant tumours as it results in least damage to the surrounding tissue compared to radiotherapy and chemotherapy. Different surgical methods are available for different types of cancers. The surgical methods used for breast cancer include lumpectomy (removal of the tumour and small healthy tissue around) and mastectomy (removal of the entire breast). There are several types of mastectomies available, depending upon the type of breast tumour [18].

The surgical procedures used for ovarian cancer include unilateral and bilateral salpingo-oophorectomy and debulking or cytoreduction [19]. The most common surgery used for endometrial cancer is a total hysterectomy.

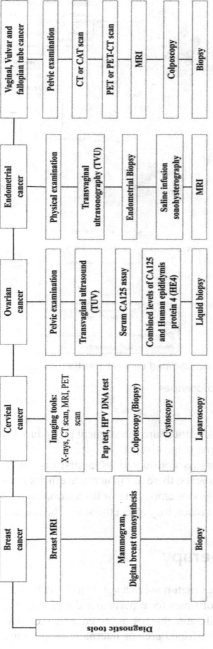

FIGURE 1.2 Tools and techniques for diagnosis of women-associated cancers.

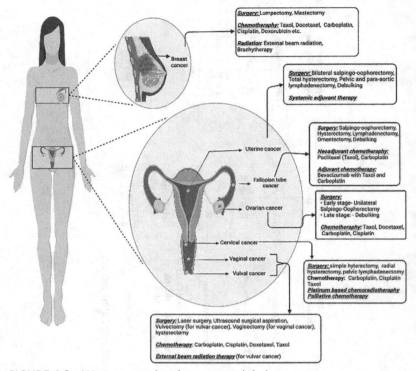

FIGURE 1.3 Women-associated cancers and their treatment.
Source: Created in Biorender.

Vulvectomy and vaginectomy are the surgical procedure used for treating vulvar and vaginal cancer, respectively.

Although surgery is considered as a first-line treatment for different women-associated cancers, there are major side effects associated with it, such as significant blood loss or clots, pain or discomfort, infections, or damage to other organs. In some cases, they affect the sexual health of women as well [20].

Radiation Therapy

Radiation therapy uses high-power energy beams such as x-rays, protons, given for specific number of times for a particular duration to eliminate cancer cells from the organ. Radiation therapy is given either externally by directing a radiation beam at an affected area or internally by placing a device filled with radioactive material inside within or near tumour. For some cancers, radiation is the only treatment required, whereas it may also be used as a part of combined multimodality treatment for other types. Some common side effects from radiation therapy includes fatigue, skin reaction, reduce bowel movements and abdominal pain. Advanced radiotherapy techniques, such as intensity-modulated RT (IMRT), have been shown to reduce treatment-related toxic effects in women [21].

Chemotherapy

Chemotherapy is a drug treatment that destroys cancer cells and stops cancer cells from growing and dividing. A chemotherapy regimen consists of a specific number of cycles given over a set period. The chemotherapeutic drugs are usually given intravenously or orally (systemic chemotherapy) whereas in certain cases it is delivered to a specific area of the body (intra-arterial, intra-cavitary and intrathecal chemotherapy). The drugs used in chemotherapy are either used alone or in combination therapies for effective treatment of cancer [22–24]. Since chemotherapeutic drugs also target normal cells, side effects ranging from mild to severe can result depending on the drug dosage. Table 1.1

TABLE 1.1   Chemotherapeutic drugs for treatment of women-associated cancers.

CHEMOTHERAPEUTIC DRUG	BRAND NAME	MODE OF ACTION	TYPE OF CANCER
Melphalan	Alkeran, Evomela	It alkylates guanine resides in DNA which leads to inhibition of DNA and RNA synthesis.	Ovarian cancer
Paclitaxel	Abraxane, Taxol	It promotes the synthesis of tubulin and inhibits the separation of microtubules, thus preventing cell cycle progression.	Cancer of the breast, cervix, endometrium, ovary, vulva and vagina
Carboplatin	Paraplatin	It inhibits DNA replication and synthesis by forming reactive platinum complex.	Cancer of the ovary, cervix, endometrium, breast, vulva and vagina

(Continued)

TABLE 1.1   (Continued)

CHEMOTHERAPEUTIC DRUG	BRAND NAME	MODE OF ACTION	TYPE OF CANCER
Docetaxel	Taxotere	It Inhibits microtubule depolymerization. Weakens the effect of antiapoptotic gene expression.	Cancer of the ovary, breast, endometrium, and vagina
Fluorouracil (5-FU)	Actikerall, Carac, Efudex, Fluoroplex, Tolak	It inhibits the activity of thymidylate synthase, thereby causing cell death in absence of thymine.	Cancer of the ovary, breast, vulva and vagina
Cyclophosphamide	Procytox	Alkylating agent, leads to cross linkage formation between strands of RNA/DNA, thus inhibiting protein synthesis.	Ovarian cancer, breast cancer
Doxorubicin	Adriamycin, Doxil, Myocet	It decelerates or prevents the growth of cancer by blocking the activity of topo-isomerase 2 enzymes.	Cancer of breast, ovary, and endometrium
Pegylated liposomal Doxorubicin	Doxil, Lipodox	Liposomes keep doxorubicin in the blood for a long time, so that most of the drug reaches the cancer cells.	Cancer of the ovary, breast, and endometrium
Vinorelbine	Navelbine	It binds microtubular proteins to the mitotic spindle, thereby preventing cell division during metaphase.	Breast cancer

CHEMOTHERAPEUTIC DRUG	BRAND NAME	MODE OF ACTION	TYPE OF CANCER
Topotecan	Hycamtin	A topoisomerase I inhibitor that it interferes with DNA replication and induces cell death.	Ovarian cancer, cervical cancer
Chlorambucil	Leukeran	It interferes with DNA replication and induces cellular apoptosis through accumulation of cytosolic p53, activating Bax, a promotor of apoptosis.	Ovarian cancer
Cisplatin	Platinol	It binds to the N7 reactive centre on purine residues and as such can cause DNA damage in cancer cells, blocking cell division and resulting in apoptotic cell death.	Cancer of the ovary, cervix, and endometrium

lists the common chemotherapeutic drugs, their brand name along with the mode of action used for different women-associated cancers.

Targeted Therapy

Since most of the advanced or recurrent women-associated cancers are associated with poor prognosis, novel therapeutic modalities to improve clinical outcomes in breast and gynaecological cancer are needed. Targeted therapy serves as a promising approach in this regard and involves treatment that targets cancer-specific genes, proteins or tissue microenvironment that contributes to cancer growth and survival [25]. Some of the molecular agents used in targeted therapy include monoclonal antibodies, small molecule inhibitors, antiangiogenic agents, poly-(ADP-ribose) polymerase (PARP) inhibitors, tumour intrinsic signalling pathway inhibitors (PI3K/AKT/mTOR) pathway inhibitors, immune checkpoint inhibitors, antibody-drug conjugates and selective estrogen receptor downregulators (SERDs) [3]. Many targeted cancer therapies have been approved by the US Food and Drug Administration (FDA) for use in cancer treatment, while others are in preclinical testing (animal studies) and in clinical trials (human studies) (Table 1.2).

TABLE 1.2   Novel targeted agents/drugs for treatment of women-associated cancers.

TARGETED AGENT/DRUG TYPE	DRUGS (FDA APPROVED)	TARGET GENE/ PATHWAY	CANCER TYPE	REFERENCE
Monoclonal antibodies	Trastuzumab, Cetuximab, Pertuzumab	EGFR and HER2 receptors	Breast cancer	[26]
Small molecule inhibitors (Tyrosine kinase inhibitors	Lapatinib Sorafenib, Sunitinib, and Pazopanib (in clinical trials)	EGFR and HER2 VEGF signalling pathways	Breast cancer Ovarian cancer	[26]
Antiangiogenic agents (Anti-VEGF antibodies)	Bevacizumab	VEGF signalling pathways	Cervical cancer Ovarian cancer	[27] [3]
Poly (ADP-ribose) polymerase (PARP) inhibitors	Olaparib, Niraparib Rucaparib	PARP-1	Ovarian cancer	[3,26]
Intrinsic signalling pathway inhibitors (PI3K/ AKT/mTOR pathway inhibitors)	Idelalisib, Alpelisib and Copanlisib Everolimus and Temsirolimus (in clinical trials)	PI3K mTOR	Breast cancer, cervical cancer, endometrial cancer	[3]
Immune checkpoint inhibitors	Anti-PD-1 antibodies (Nivolumab, Pembrolizumab), and anti-PD-L1 antibodies	PD-1 pathway	Cervical cancer, endometrial cancer	[3]

TARGETED AGENT/DRUG TYPE	DRUGS (FDA APPROVED)	TARGET GENE/ PATHWAY	CANCER TYPE	REFERENCE
	(Atezolizumab, Durvalumab, Avelumab) (in clinical trials) Pembrolizumab			
Antibody-drug conjugates	Mirvetuximab Soravtansine (in clinical trials)	Folate receptor α (FRα)	Ovarian cancer, cervical cancer	[3]
	Tisotumab vedotin (HuMax-TF) (in clinical trials)	Tissue factor (TF)	Cervical cancer	
Selective estrogen receptor downregulators (SERDs)	Fulvestrant	Estrogen receptors	Breast cancer	[3]

Immunotherapy

Immunotherapy is the cancer treatment that uses body defences to fight cancer. The immunotherapy drugs include CART cell therapy, immune checkpoint inhibitors, monoclonal antibodies, treatment vaccines, and immunomodulators (Table 1.2). Currently, along with traditional treatment, new advanced treatment strategies are used for the treatment of women-associated cancers.

CONCLUSION

The overall burden of women-associated cancer incidence and mortality is rapidly growing worldwide despite recent advances in cancer treatments. Among women, breast cancer has the highest incidence and mortality rate, followed by cervical, endometrial and ovarian cancers. Increasing public awareness among women on the possible cancer risk factors and implementation of specific primary (vaccine) and secondary (screening strategies) prevention measures might reduce an individual's risk of cancer mortality. Although current treatments like radiotherapy, chemotherapy, targeted and immunotherapy are effective in treating the disease, still there remains an unmet need to find novel and efficient therapies which can alleviate critical side effects caused by conventional treatments. With advancements in clinical cancer research and medicine, new treatment modalities like hormone-based therapy, gene therapy, stem cell therapy and dendritic cell-based immunotherapy are developed for diagnosis, and treatment of breast and gynaecological cancer in women. When used along with conventional therapies, these reduce the chances of cancer reoccurrence and have been associated with best patient outcomes.

REFERENCES

1. Lindsey A Torre et al. Cancer Epidemiol Biomarkers Prev. (2017), PMID: 28223433.
2. Hyuna Sung et al. CA Cancer J Clin. (2021), PMID: 33538338.
3. Qiao Wang et al. Signal Transduct Target Ther. (2020), PMID: 32728057.
4. Ye-seul Kim et al. Oncol Rep. (2015), PMID: 25760693.
5. AD Waldman et al. Nature Rev Immunol. (2020), PMID: 32433532.
6. A Awan et al. Curr Oncol. (2018), PMID: 30111969.
7. An Coosemans et al. Oncoimmunology. (2013), PMID: 24501688.
8. Paul A Cohen et al. Lancet. (2019), PMID: 30638582.
9. J Ferlay et al. Int J Cancer. (2001), PMID: 11668491.
10. DM Parkin et al. CA Cancer J Clin. (2005), PMID: 15761078.
11. J Ferlay et al. Int J Cancer. (2010), PMID: 21351269.
12. J Ferlay et al. Int J Cancer. (2015), PMID: 25220842.
13. F Bray et al. CA Cancer J. Clin. (2018), PMID: 30207593.
14. AA Onitilo et al. Clin Med Res. (2009), PMID: 19574486.
15. Emma J Crosbie et al. Lancet. (2013), PMID: 23618600.
16. Simon A Gayther, et al. Curr Opin Genet Dev. (2010), PMID: 20456938.
17. T Karlsson et al. Cancer Res. (2021), PMID: 33334812.
18. A Covens et al. Cancer: Interdiscip I J Am Cancer Soc. (1999), PMID: 10590368.
19. UA Matulonis et al. Nat. Rev. Dis. Primers. (2016), PMID: 27558151.
20. RN Pauls et al. Int. J. Impot. (2010), PMID: 20072131.
21. X Li, S Kitpanit et al. JAMA Network Open. (2021), PMID: 34143193.
22. FA Fisusi et al. Pharm Nanotechnol. (2019), PMID: 30666921.
23. B Orr et al. Hematol/Oncol Clin. (2018), PMID: 30390767.
24. J Rahaman et al. Mt Sinai J Med. (2009), PMID: 20014427
25. M Padma et al. BioMedicinevol. (2015), PMID: 26613930.
26. Partha Basu et al. Int J Gynaecol Obstet. (2018), PMID: 30306576.
27. MW Jackson et al. OncoTargets Ther. (2014), PMID: 24876784.

Cancer Drugs and Treatment Formulations for Women-Associated Cancers

2

Reetika Arora and Pawan K. Maurya

Contents

DOI: 10.1201/9781003260172-2

15

INTRODUCTION

Cancer is a serious public health issue across the world [1]. As per the World Health Organization (WHO) statistics for 2019, cancer is the primary or second leading cause of death before the age of 70 in 112 of 183 countries, and ranks third or fourth in another 23 [2]. The worldwide burden of cancer and mortality is on the rise; this is due to changes in the prevalence and distribution of the primary cancer risk factors, some of which are linked to socioeconomic development, as well as population expansion and ageing [3]. Traditionally, women have been found to be less affected than their male counterparts by cancer. As reported by the National Cancer Institute, one out of every three women, and one out of every two males, will be diagnosed with cancer at some time in their lives [4]. The cancer detection is frequently linked to genealogy of the disease, lifestyle choices, or environmental influences. While it may be impossible to manage family history or the entire environment, healthy lifestyle practices such as a balanced diet, regular physical activity, nutritional treatment, and quitting smoking may all be controlled [5].

Women are more presumably than men to survive the disorder. According to data by GLOBOCAN 2020 (Global Cancer Observatory), breast cancer is the most common cancer in women (11.7% of all cases) and the leading cause of cancer-related death (6.9%) [6] in terms of incidence and mortality; colorectal and lung cancers come in second and third, respectively [3]. Malignancies of the endometrium, cervix, skin and ovary are also among the most often diagnosed cancers in women. In contrast to males, the worldwide variety of widely diagnosed and the leading cause of death on the basis of gender, the most commonly diagnosed cancers in women were found to be breast cancer (159 countries) and cervical cancer (23 of the remaining 26 countries) [3]. Breast and cervical cancer are the top causes of cancer mortality in 110 and 36 nations, respectively, while lung cancer is the leading cause of death in 25 countries [7].

Breast Cancer

Breast cancer is a result of breast tissue modification and uncontrolled multiplication, leading to the formation of mass or lump. The lobules or tubes that connect the lobules to the nipple are where most breast cancers begin [8]. The growth of a firm, painless lump that may expand is the most common physical symptom. Symptoms such as breast heaviness or soreness, ulceration, erythema, thickness, and inflammation may occur. Modulations of the nipple, retraction or scaliness, and spontaneous discharge from the nipple, particularly bloody discharge, may be seen [9]. Breast cancer can sometimes spread to the lymph nodes in the under-arm, causing swelling or lumps [10]. Previous history, extensive family history, and genetic susceptibility (abnormal genes, BRCA1 and BRCA2), alcohol consumption, being overweight, hormonal causes, as well as lifestyle and dietary factors, along with environmental triggers are the leading causes of breast cancer [5]. African American women under the age of 40 are twice as likely as white women of the same age to develop breast cancer. Another distinction of breast cancer is that African American and Hispanic women are more likely to be diagnosed in the disease's severe and advanced stages. The need for more effective breast cancer remedies is highlighted by these inconsistencies [11].

Gynaecologic Cancer

When cancer is diagnosed in a woman's reproductive organs, it is called gynaecologic cancer. The five most frequent types of gynaecologic cancer are cervical, ovarian, uterine, vaginal, and vulvar cancer [12]. (There is a sixth type of gynaecologic cancer, fallopian tube cancer, which is extremely uncommon). Cervical cancer is the only cancer that has screening tests that can detect the disease at an early stage, when treatment is most effective [4].

Ovarian Cancer

Cancer of the ovaries is the fifth leading cause of death among women in the United States. Serbia has the highest rate of incidence of ovarian cancer followed by Brunei in 2018, according to World Cancer Research Fund International. The American Cancer Society further predicts 21,410 new cases to be diagnosed in United States. While it accounts for only 3% of all the cancers that affect women, it is multifactorial.

Cervical Cancer

It is cancer of the cervix mainly caused by the human papillomavirus (HPV) infection or the result of exposure to the drug diethylstilbestrol (DES). Other factors, like taking oral contraceptives over a long duration and smoking, also predispose a woman to cervical cancer. Examining the health history and physical exam, the Pap test, pelvic exam, HPV test, endocervical curettage, colposcopy and biopsy are some of the prognosis tests available. If cancer is detected, diagnostic tests like CT scan, PET scan, MRI, ultrasound, cystoscopy or laparoscopy can be performed to determine the stage of cervical cancer.

Vaginal Cancer

Vaginal cancer is of two types: (1) squamous cell carcinoma and (2) adenocarcinoma. Squamous cell vaginal cancer grows slowly and generally stays close to the vaginal area, although it can also move to the lungs, liver and bones. The most frequent kind of vaginal cancer is this one, whereas adenocarcinoma is a kind of cancer that starts in glandular cells. Glandular cells in the vaginal lining produce and discharge fluids like mucus. Adenocarcinoma is more likely to spread to the lungs and lymph nodes. Older age and having HPV infection are the risk factors of developing vaginal cancer.

Uterine Cancer (Endometrial Cancer)

Uterine cancer was shown to be responsible for 7% of all cancer cases and 4% of female cancer deaths [5]. Uterine cancer affects one out of every 36 women. It is cancer of the uterine lining, the endometrium, which makes it more prevalent than cervical or ovarian malignancies. Unlike cervical cancer, it is not a gynaecological malignancy caused by HPV. Hormonal imbalances, notably estrogen, play a key role in the development of uterine cancer, which, like breast cancer, feeds on estrogen. Taking estrogen after menopause, birth control pills, a higher number of menstrual cycles (over a lifetime), previous or current use of tamoxifen for breast cancer, infertility, obesity and having polycystic ovarian syndrome are all factors that can alter hormone levels and increase the risk of uterine cancer [5].

Colorectal Cancer

Colorectal cancer starts in either the colon or rectum. Being overweight or obese, inactivity, having a diet high in red and processed meats, smoking, heavy alcohol use, age, and a personal or family history of colorectal cancer or polyps are all risk factors for colorectal cancer [13].

Thyroid Cancer

Thyroid cancer has grown substantially in prevalence over the last three decades, and it is currently the fastest growing disease in women. According to the most recent American Cancer Society predictions, there will be roughly 43,800 new cases of thyroid cancer in the United States in 2022 (11,860 in men and 31,940 in women) (12,150 in men and 32,130 in women) [14]. Thyroid cancer claims the lives of over 2,230 deaths from thyroid cancer (1,070 men and 1,160 women) people each year (approx. 1,050 men and 1,150 women) www. cancer.org; ACS Journal; seer.cancer.gov. Thyroid cancer has an unknown origin, although it may be caused by a mix of hereditary and environmental factors. While some people have no signs or symptoms, others may have a bulge in the neck. Surgery, hormone therapy, radioactive iodine, radiation and, in certain circumstances, chemotherapy are all effective treatments.

CANCER TREATMENT AND MANAGEMENT

There are multiple approaches for management of cancer depending upon the stage of cancer. Some of the approaches are as follows:

Surgery might be recommended in order to remove the cancer-affected tissue/organ, hormonal therapy using tamoxifen drugs which blocks the estrogen receptor in tumour, radiation therapy deploys high-energy rays to prevent chance of recurrence, however, there are multiple reported side effects to this including fatigue, numbness, and damage to nerves to name a few.

Chemotherapy is another type of widely accepted method of cancer treatment and management. The side effects reported, however, are too many, including hair loss, nausea, neuropathy, cardiomyopathy and many more.

Immunotherapy is aimed for stimulating the immune system for destroying tumours. In the case of breast cancer, atezolizumab and pembrolizumab are the two immunotherapeutic drugs approved by the FDA for treatment in metastatic triple negative breast cancer. Both of them are immune checkpoint inhibitors.

Natural compounds, which are chemical molecules generated from biological organisms, can promote apoptosis and cell cycle arrest, which can inhibit carcinogenesis and reverse cancer growth. They affect tumour cells through influencing cell death mechanisms, including extrinsic and intrinsic apoptosis and autophagy [13]. In these processes, these substances inhibit the growth of cancer cells without causing severe harm to normal cells [15]. Some of the compounds being used in cancer treatment are quercetin (QC), an anticancer, antioxidant, antitumour and anti-inflammatory flavanol [2] found in a variety of vegetables and fruits as well as wine, tea, and coffee [12], which belongs to the flavonoid group of polyphenols. QC inhibits the synthesis of anti-apoptotic proteins like survivin, Bcl-xL, and Bcl-2, while raising the expression of pro-apoptotic proteins like Bad and Bax to urge cancer cells to die [11]. Natural chemicals are increasingly being evaluated for application in clinical research due to their anticancer and apoptotic properties, as well as their low toxicity.

Curcumin (CUR), the main component in turmeric, regulates the creation of a number of proteins essential for cell survival and proliferation, including inflammatory cytokines and enzymes, transcription factors and gene products [16]. This polyphenol derivative also inhibits angiogenesis and tumour metastasis while promoting apoptosis [1]. CUR stops human BrCa cells from proliferating by blocking nuclear factor kappaB activation, which has been associated to cancer cell survival, growth and metastasis [15]. In BT-474 and SK-BR-3 cells, CUR also suppresses MAPK and NF-B [11,15]. Anti-apoptotic proteins like BCL-xL and BCL-2, as well as proliferative and metastatic proteins like cyclin-D1 and c-Myc, vascular endothelial growth factor, and intercellular adhesion molecule-1 [14], are all inhibited by this drug. CUR inhibits tumour growth and reduces the number of viable cells in the BrCa cell line MDAMB-231, indicating that it has therapeutic potential for BrCa therapy [11]. Silibinin, thymoquinone, garcinol, genistein, diosgenin, honokiol, resveratrol, and tetrandrine are some of the other natural compounds which have promising potential to treat cancer.

NANOTECHNOLOGY: THE WAY FORWARD

Nanomedicine is an essential factor of nanotechnology; it deals with the extremely specialized intervention of medicine at the molecular level in illness prevention, diagnosis, and therapy. Nano- and microscale drug delivery technologies have shown to be extremely helpful in the creation of therapeutically effective formulations. Nanodrug delivery systems are developing in the market for the treatment of different illnesses, including cancer [4,15].

Nanoparticles offer the added benefit of increasing the solubility of medicines, reduced dosage and toxicity, improved cellular absorption, and so forth. Because of their tiny size, these are rapidly absorbed by tumour cells and efficiently encapsulate hydrophobic molecules. The other benefits of nanotechnology in cancer treatment include precise medication targeting via active or passive targeting, reduced systemic toxicity, controlled-release drug delivery, the ability to mix several medicines for successful therapy, better bioavailability of the cancer drug, and so on. The US Food and Drug Administration (FDA) has authorized nanomaterials for diagnosis and treatment of breast cancer. Thus, nanotechnology seems to be way forward for future cancer trials and treatment.

Liposomes: The prototypical nanoscale drug delivery methods are liposomes and other lipid-based drug delivery systems [17]. Recent trials and research outcomes, have given lot of attention to liposomes as one of the suitable pharmaceutical drug carriers. Liposomes are self-assembling entities consisting of a bilayer membrane surrounding an aqueous inner chamber. When it comes to developing liposomes, there is a lot of flexibility in terms of composition, size, and drug release qualities, for example. Several components govern features such as elimination half-lives, permeability, biodistribution, and targeted selectivity in liposomal nanoparticles, which are meant to be multifunctional [16–17]. Commercially available lipids for liposome NPs include cholesterol, phosphatidylcholine, phosphatidylethanolamine, and phosphatidylserine [18]. A study by Slingerland et al. found out increased antitumour efficacy and reduced toxicity when studying liposomal anticancer drugs available in the market for breast cancer, ovarian cancer, and Kaposi's sarcoma [8,17]. However, while liposomal anticancer drugs have evolved over the years, developing novel liposome formulations building up on the available textual information and also conducting phased trials should be the way forward.

Metal-organic frameworks (MOFs) are porous NPs made up of a metal ion and an organic linker or spacer in a variety of hybrid configurations [7,18]. MOFs have the potential for regulated drug release due to their large surface area and varied pore size. MOFs, on the other hand, must be scaled down to the nanoscale in order to be useful as anticancer drug carriers in vivo [10]. For nanocarrier production, biocompatible and biodegradable polymers such as polylactic acid (PLA) esters and their copolymers with glycolic acid (PLGA), poly(-caprolactone), polyglutamic acid, and poly (alkyl cyanoacrylate) have lately acquired popularity [6,10,18].

CONCLUSION

While there is a lot of research going on in nanomedicine, the lack of standard protocols for characterization of nanocarriers and nanodrugs, toxicity, physical, chemical, and biological instability, disease heterogeneity, and irregular in vivo behaviour of NPs often limits the desired outcomes, resulting in NP failure in late-phase clinical trials. To minimize clinical trial failure, it is necessary to study cancer heterogeneity and inherent features of NPs in order to correctly alter them for enhanced stability, biocompatibility, and consistent in vivo behaviour. The data acquired from research trials needs to be corroborated with multidisciplinary approaches to overcome the challenges and design an integrated system for meeting the demanding needs of an effective management of cancer.

CONFLICTS OF INTEREST/ COMPETING INTERESTS

The authors report no conflicts of interest.

REFERENCES

1. K. Terlikowska et al. *Advances in Hygiene and Experimental Medicine* (2014). PMID: 24864107.
2. A. Patra et al. *International Journal of Nanomedicine* (2018). PMID: 29844670.
3. Lu Chen et al. *American Association for Cancer Research* (2015). DOI: 10.1158/1055-9965.EPI-15-0293.
4. K. Park. *Journal of Controlled Release* (2008). PMID: 17532520.
5. Millimouno et al. *Cancer Prevention Research* (2014). DOI: 10.1158/1940-6207. CAPR-14-0136.
6. E. Calzoni et al. *Journal of Functional Biomaterials* (2019). DOI: 10.3390/jfb10010004
7. D. Eom et al. *Journal of Nanoscience and Nanotechnology* (2015). DOI: 10.1166/jnn.2015.10368
8. M. Slingerland. et al. *Drug Discovery Today* (2012). DOI: 10.1016/j.drudis.2011.09.015
9. S. B. Diwate et al. *Journal of Pharmaceutical Research International* (2020) DOI: 10.9734/jpri/2020/v32i3630991.
10. N. Bhardwaj et al. *Toxicology Research* (2018). DOI: 10.1039/c8tx00087e
11. Hyuna Sung et al. *ACS* (2021). DOI: 10.3322/caac.21660
12. D. Liu et al. *Journal of Breast Cancer* (2013). DOI: 10.4048/jbc.2013.16.2.133
13. J. M. Manouchehri et al. *Breast Cancer (Auckl)* (2018). DOI: 10.1177/1178223417749855

14. B. B. Aggarwal et al. *Clin Cancer Research* (2005). DOI: 10.1158/1078-0432.
    CCR-05-1192
15. S. Bimonte et al. *BioMed Research International* (2015). DOI:
    10.1155/2015/878134
16. T. M. Allen et al. *Anti-cancer Agents in Medicinal Chemistry* (2006). DOI:
    10.2174/187152006778699121
17. T. N. Aung et al. *International Journal of Molecular Sciences* (2017). DOI:
    10.3390/ijms18030656.
18. M. Arnold et al. *The Lancet Oncology* (2019). DOI: 10.1016/S1470-2045
    (19)30456-5.

Imaging as an Important Tool for Diagnosis of Breast Cancer

3

Priyanka Mudaliar, Shafina Siddiqui,
Sangeeta Ballav, Narrayan Raam Shankar,
Soumya Basu and Jyotirmoi Aich

Contents

DOI: 10.1201/9781003260172-3

REQUIREMENTS FOR BREAST IMAGING

Breast imaging is considered a significant non-invasive modality for evaluation of the breast for any kind of physiologic variations with benign or malignant tumours. Technical advancements for breast cancer detection restrain their usage due to failure of thorough examination of the disease in terms of shape, size and appearance. Therefore, imaging modality implies a powerful technique that provides early detection with successive follow-up. There are various imaging techniques available that help to profile the advanced staging of breast cancer. Table 3.1 summarizes the advantages and disadvantages of individual techniques. These breast imaging modalities detect the breast cancer metastases according to disease stages and generate images with increased image sharpness and high specificity.

TABLE 3.1   Advantages and disadvantages of different breast cancer modalities.

BREAST CANCER MODALITIES	ADVANTAGES	DISADVANTAGES	REFERENCES
Mammography	Reduces mortality rate about 20%–40% Provides early detection	High false positives Induction of radiation dose in highly sensitive breast tissue Over-diagnosis	[1–2]

BREAST CANCER MODALITIES	ADVANTAGES	DISADVANTAGES	REFERENCES
DBT	Increased cancer detection by 15%–30% Low false positives Decreased recall rate by 15%–20%	Increased radiation dose by 20%	[1,6]
CEDM	Highly sensitive (93%–100%) High specificity (87%)	Probable allergic reactions from iodinated contrast agent Increased radiation dose by 20%–80%	[1,2,9]
CTLM	No use of ionizing radiation Highly sensitive and specificity	Time-consuming and complicated Not approved by FDA	[11–12]
SPECT	Highly sensitive (96.4%)	Low specificity (59.5%) High radiation exposure High false negatives	[2,13]
PET	High resolution High sensitivity and specificity	High exposure to radiation Costly	[2–3]
ABUS	Better breast cancer detection rate (89.9%)	Lesions may be missed if present in a peripheral location	[14–15]
CEUS	Very high sensitivity	Lack of availability of this modality in clinical practice	[17]
AVBS	Saves time	Low specificity (52.8%)	[18]
3D ultrasound	High specificity	Not prevalent in clinical practice due to being relatively new	[19–20]
Doppler sonography	High sensitivity and specificity (both 88%)	Not easy to distinguish between benign and malignant tumours	[21]
Tissue elasticity imaging	Operator independence, reproducibility	Expensive equipment	[22–23]

(*Continued*)

TABLE 3.1   (Continued)

BREAST CANCER MODALITIES	ADVANTAGES	DISADVANTAGES	REFERENCES
Stress elastography	Suitable for quantitative analyses Good reproducibility	Expensive equipment	[24]
MRI	Does not use ionizing radiation	High risk to patients Possibility of false positive results Does not show calcium deposits	[25–26]
DWI	Short scanning time	Produces lower image quality and artifacts	[29–30]
MRE	Non-invasive	Requires co-operation by patients due to its breath-hold technique	[31–32]
MRS	Robust and reproducible	Unable to detect low levels of metabolites	[34]
Optical imaging	Easily accessible	Less sensitive and specific	[36]

IMAGING MODALITIES

X-ray/Laser Imaging Technologies

Conventional Mammography

Mammography is a two-dimensional (2D) imaging method that focuses on morphological characteristics of breast cancer [1]. In this technique, the breast tissue is compressed between two firm parallel plates. A low energy x-ray (25–32 kVp) is used to create 2D radiographic images of these tissues which are either recorded on a film or saved instantly on a computer [2]. The BI-RADS (Breast Imaging Reporting and Data System), formed by the American College of Radiology, specifies precise terminology for reporting breast radiography [3]. The American College of Radiology along with other institutes also recommended annual mammograms for women starting at age of 40 [4].

Digital Breast Tomosynthesis (DBT)

DBT is a relatively new advancement in digital mammography that provides seemingly three-dimensional (3D) images of the breast, hence enhancing sensitivity and specificity [5]. In this technique, the x-ray tube spin around a limited angle (15–60 degrees) from the pressed breast tissue, producing 3D breast images which are generated by exposing the breast tissue frequently at distinct angles and reconstructing the images as half-millimetre sections [2]. DBT is endorsed by the National Comprehensive Cancer Network (NCCN) as an admissible modality for breast cancer screening [6]. It is gradually being utilized as a replacement for digital mammography, for which it was used as a supplement before [7].

Contrast-Enhanced Digital Mammography (CEDM)

CEDM utilizes intravenous administration of an iodinated contrast agent via an injection prior to a mammography examination [8–9]. The mammography examination is performed around 2 minutes after the administration of the contrast agent. During compression, the apparatus acquires two images: a low-energy picture and a high-energy picture. The lower energy picture is utilized for regular mammography, whilst the higher energy picture is post-handled to produce images that at most show the intensifying tumours [10]. For image interpretation, there is currently no CEDM-specific BI-RADS terminology. As a result, low-energy images are evaluated using the BI-RADS mammography terminology, and recombined images are evaluated using the BI-RADS MRI terminology [3].

Computed Tomography Laser Mammography (CTLM)

CTLM is an optical imaging technology used to test for breast cancer in women under the age of 40 having dense breasts [10–11]. CTLM assesses tissue optical characteristics using near-infrared light propagation through the tissue. For each wavelength, various tissue factors can affect dispersion and absorption properties [11]. Imaging Diagnostic Systems, Inc. (IDSI, United States) owns the CTLM trademark for its optical tomographic technology for female breast imaging. It was designated as a Class III medical device in 2011. It is now being evaluated by the Food and Drug Administration (FDA) in the United States and is being proposed as a mammography adjunct [12].

Imaging With Gamma Rays

Single-Photon Emission Computed Tomography (SPECT)

SPECT is a radiology imaging diagnostic technology which utilizes gamma rays [13]. In SPECT, ^{99m}Tc (a radiopharmaceutical) is taken up by activated mitochondria in malignant breast cells after injection. Gamma rays with an energy of around 140 keV are emitted and collected in a huge planar gamma detector underneath the compressed breast [2]. Combining SPECT with CT (computed tomography) enhances the accuracy of breast cancer diagnosis [13].

Positron Emission Tomography (PET)

PET imaging modality is a molecular tomographic technique that is used for quantifying the metabolic and physiological activity of cells [2]. PET involves injecting a small amount of radioisotope like 18F FDG (fluorodeoxyglucose), a positron emitter radiotracer, into the patient. The radionuclide is then spread throughout the body, and once it decays, it releases a positron in just about any random direction. When a positron collides with an electron within the body while travelling, the two particles disintegrate and create two 511 keV gamma rays. To identify the two gamma rays in tandem, positron emission mammography (PEM) camera is utilized [3]. PET in conjunction with CT has a higher sensitivity for detecting tumours than traditional imaging [1].

Imaging With Ultrasound Wave

Sonography

Sonography (ultrasound) used to be one of the main diagnostic methods for the diagnosis and/or early detection of breast cancer and other diseases of the breast. Nowadays, however, it has largely fallen out of grace in favour of more modern techniques involving x-rays, gamma rays, and other modern imaging mechanisms. However, since this technique has been around for quite a while, it remains commonplace in many regions.

Automated Breast Ultrasound (ABUS)

ABUS are more recent additions to the market, used mainly for breast imaging [14]. The instrument is used on the patient lying in a supine position. A computer-guided machine arm acquires the images through the attached transducers. It has been reported that there is a significant improvement observed in the detection of breast lesions with the use of ABUS with a mammogram [15].

Contrast-Enhanced Ultrasound (CEUS)

CEUS implies the application of intravenous contrast agents consisting of microbubbles/nanobubbles of gas and using acoustic pressure to detect lesions using ultrasound. The ultrasound beam leads to oscillation of these microbubbles compressed with positive pressure whereas expand on negative pressure [16]. The most significant feature of CEUS is that the procedure can differentiate between benign and malignant tumours. This feature dramatically helps in reducing the number of core-cut biopsies performed in benign lesions [17].

Automated Breast Volume Scanner (AVBS)

AVBS possess a high frequency of about 5–14 MHz, which is employed to patients in the prone position [18]. The main components of AVBS are a touchscreen, a flexible arm with the transducer at the end, and a 3D workstation. The ACUSON S2000 (Siemens) is vividly utilized due to its consistency and reproducible results.

Three-Dimensional Ultrasound

3D ultrasound involves the conversion of standard 2D images obtained from ultrasound into a quantitative dataset, which is then reviewed retrospectively [19]. The technique has gained greater attention due to the production of high-quality images with illustrative breast density. Depending on this property, it is leading to adjuncts to mammography [20]. Its use is not prevalent currently, due to the method being relatively new. However, with time, we can expect its usage to increase, compared to its other ultrasound imaging counterparts.

Doppler Sonography

Doppler sonography is an indispensable tool that is extensively used to study breast tumours. It has become an integral and fundamental part of breast ultrasound [21]. The tool consists of a handheld device, a transducer, which moves lightly over the skin above a blood vessel that ultimately produces sound waves amplified through a microphone. These sound waves reflect the solid objects, such as blood cells and helps detecting any physiological changes such as angiogenesis.

Tissue-Elasticity Imaging (TEI)

Tissue-elasticity imaging is a quantitative method conventionally used for observing the stiffness of tissue. The images obtained through this tool contain either an image of estimated elastic modulus or an image of strain in response to force [22]. Broadly, tissue-elasticity imaging techniques are categorized into static ultrasound elastography which consists of strain imaging and dynamic ultrasound elastography which includes shear wave and acoustic radiation force impulse imaging [23].

Stress Elastography

Stress elastography is one of the elastography techniques which involves non-invasive examination of tissue mechanical properties. The images obtained are measured through specialized imaging modes which detects tissue stiffness in response to shear waves. Shear waves are generated either by putting an external mechanical vibration or acoustic radiation force impulses [24].

Imaging Using Magnetic Field

Magnetic Resonance Imaging (MRI)

MRI is known to be efficient and non-invasive technique, used for medical investigation and imaging, over 30 years [25]. It uses a magnetic field to create the cross-sectional images of breast tissues by measuring the movement of hydrogen nuclei (protons) present in fat and water [3,26]. Interestingly, machine learning techniques have been applied in MRI for segregating the breast tissues and detection of various subtypes of cancer [27].

Diffusion-Weighted Imaging (DWI)

DWI captures the random motion of microscopic water protons in the body and provides both quantitative and qualitative information regarding motion patterns [28]. In some conditions, this random motion is disturbed and results in the change of the motion in the affected area. This strategy is exploited for imaging the internal physiology [29]. Nowadays, DWI has also been used in association with MRI in the field of oncology and in the management of musculoskeletal problems such as bone cancer and rheumatologic diseases [30].

Magnetic Resonance Elastography (MRE)

MRE is a non-invasive method that quantitatively assess the mechanical properties of tissues and analyses stiffness of the tissue by the propagation of mechanical waves with the help of MRI technique [31]. A group of researchers have reported the nature of breast cancer tissues as harder and stiffer compared to the healthy fibro-glandular tissue [32].

Magnetic Resonance Spectroscopy (MRS)

MRS is an in vivo technique used for evaluating the biochemical nature of the human diseases [33]. It is carried out at high magnetic field strength, approximately 11–14 Tesla on body fluids, cell extracts and tissue samples, to draw anatomical as well as functional information [34]. Recently, researchers and clinicians have been using Proton MRS (^{1}H MRS) to deeply analyse and monitor breast cancer development through measuring choline, phosphocholine and glycerol phosphocholine levels in the body [35].

Non-ionizing Radiation

Optical Imaging

Optical imaging provides the optical properties of breast cancer tissues with the use of propagation of light [36]. A near-infrared range (NIR) light is used, which is transmitted by optical imaging devices through the breast and results in absorbing and scattering of light by tissue components. The remaining light is detected and recorded by detectors that are used for visualize the images [36–37].

Breast Microwave Imaging

Microwave imaging is primarily used for early-stage detection of breast cancer [38]. The underlying principle lies in assessing the differences in dielectric properties between a normal and cancerous tissues of breast [39–40]. In this method, microwaves are allowed to reflect or scatter from breast tissues and the resultant waves are used for generation of images that shows the difference between malignant and healthy tissues [41–42]. The Galway University Hospital in Ireland is one of the few hospitals in the world which have installed this imaging technique [42].

REFERENCES

1. Leiner T, Carr JC. Diagn Interv Imag. 2019. PMID: 32096929.
2. Heywang-Köbrunner SH et al. Breast Care. 2011. PMID: 21779225.
3. Iranmakani S et al. Egypt J Radiol Nucl Med. 2020. DOI: 10.1186/s43055-020-00175-5.
4. Friedewald SM. Cancer Treat Res. 2018. PMID: 29349756.
5. Comstock CE et al. JAMA—J Am Med Assoc. 2020. PMID: 32096852.
6. Zackrisson S et al. Lancet Oncol. 2018. PMID: 303228170.
7. Sree SV et al. World J Clin Oncol. 2011. PMID: 21611093.
8. Baltzer PAT et al. Memo. 2017. PMID: 28989543.
9. Ghaderi KF et al. RadioGraphics. 2019. PMID: 31697627.
10. Jalalian A et al. J Digit Imag. 2017. PMID: 28429195.
11. Poellinger A et al. Acad Radiol. 2008. PMID: 19000871.
12. Pesapane F et al. Insights Imag. 2020. PMID: 32548731.
13. Krzhivitskii PI et al. Nucl Med Commun. 2019. PMID: 30507749.
14. Berg WA et al. Radiology. 2004. PMID: 15486214.
15. Elkhalek A et al. Egypt J Radiol Nucl Med. 2019. DOI: 10.1186/s43055-019-0051-6.
16. Czarniecki et al. Radiopaedia.org. 2014. DOI: 10.53347/rID-27413.
17. Janu E et al. BMC Med Imag. 2020. DOI: 10.1186/s12880-020-00467-2.
18. Wöhrle NK et al. Radiologe. 2010. PMID: 20949253.
19. Morgan M et al. Radiopaedia.org. 2015. DOI: 10.53347/rID-33139.
20. Vourtsis A. Diagn Interv Imag. 2019. PMID: 30962169.
21. Horvath E. et al. Revista Chilena de Radiología. 2011.
22. Garra BS. Ultrasound Q. 2007. PMID: 18090836.
23. Imtiaz S. Appl Radiol. 2018.
24. Sigrist RMS et al. Theranostics. 2017. PMID: 28435467.
25. Fatahi M et al. Curr Radiol Rep. 2017. DOI: 10.1007/s40134–017–0216-x.
26. Salem DS et al. J Thoracic Dis. 2013. DOI: 10.3978/j.issn.2072–1439.2013.05.02.
27. Chan HP et al. Br J Radiol. 2020. PMID: 31742424.
28. Baliyan V et al. World J. Cardiol. 2016. DOI: 10.4329/wjr.v8.i9.785.
29. Chilla GS et al. Quant Imaging Med Surgery. 2015. PMID: 26029644.
30. Lee K et al. J Clin Orthop Trauma. 2019. DOI: 10.1016/j.jcot.2019.05.018.
31. Serai SD et al. Radiology. 2017. PMID: 1000000221.
32. Lima ZS et al. Open Access Macedonian J Med Sci. 2019. DOI: 10.3889/oamjms.2019.171.
33. Ehman RL et al. J. Magn. Reson Imaging. 2012. PMID: 22987755.
34. Tognarelli JM et al. J Clin Exp Hepatol. 2015. DOI: 10.1016/j.jceh.2015.10.006.
35. Nelson MT et al. Semin Breast Dis. 2008. DOI: 10.1053/j.sembd.2008.03.004.
36. Herranz M et al. J Oncol. 2012. DOI: 10.1155/2012/863747.
37. Hadjipanayis CG et al. Semin Oncol. 2011. PMID: 21362519.
38. Arranz A et al. Front Pharmacol. 2015. DOI: 10.3389/fphar.2015.00189.

39. Kwon S et al. Int J Biomed Imag. 2016. DOI: 10.1155/2016/5054912.
40. Moloney BM et al. Acad Radiol. 2021. DOI: https://doi.org/10.1016/j.acra.2021.06.012.
41. Modiri A et al. Med Phys. 2017. PMID: 28976568.
42. Fasoula A et al. Diagnostics. 2018. DOI: 10.3390/diagnostics8030053.

Use of Immunotherapy in Gynaecological and Breast Cancer

4

Showket Hussain, Sandeep Sisodiya, Vishakha Kasherwal, Sonam Tulsyan and Asiya Khan

Contents

DOI: 10.1201/9781003260172-4

INTRODUCTION

Several types of cancers have been detected in women worldwide. In the year 2020, 9,227,484 new cases of female cancers were observed, with breast cancer alone accounting for 2,261,419 new cases [1]. Even the cancer mortality rate across the world is increasing every year. The gynaecologic cancers such as cervical, vulvar, endometrial, vaginal and ovarian/tubal/peritoneal start in the female reproductive organs. According to the GLOBOCAN 2021, gynaecological cancers, including breast cancer, are known to produce maximum mortality rates with a high risk of incidence depending on geographical location. The risk factors found to be associated with gynaecologic cancers and breast cancer are most commonly obesity, a sedentary lifestyle, hormonal imbalance, late childbirth and the use of contraceptives [2–3], except in the case of cervical cancer, which is found to be highly associated with the infection of high-risk (HR) human papillomavirus (HPV) [4].

The recent advancement in the field of tumour immunology is crucial in understanding the communication that takes place among immune cells in the tumour microenvironment. In 1957, Burnet and Thomas hypothesized the idea that tumour cells have the self-capacity to produce distinct antigenic targets that are recognized as foreign molecules by the host immune system, which leads to the elimination of tumour cells [5–6]. Therefore, immunotherapeutic approaches are aimed to achieve better treatment response against cancer cells by using immune checkpoint inhibitors (ICIs) and the selection of antigen in vaccine-based approaches to enhance T-cell proliferation through a mechanism known as adoptive cellular therapy (ACT). One of the widely studied ICI is programmed death-ligand 1 (PDL-1), a cell surface protein that is known to be expressed on tumour cells. This protein interacts with the receptors present on the immune cells, allowing tumour progression. ICI targets the PDL-1 in such a way that PDL-1 is blocked, which in turn inhibits the further downstream signalling processes. Due to its mode of action, ICI monotherapy has proven to be highly effective in several tumours [7–8]. Another very important ICI is cytotoxic T lymphocyte antigen-4 (CTL-4), which has two conventional pathways for T-cell activation [9]. The first signal is during the recognition of antigen via T-cell receptor (TCR), and the second signal is generated upon merging B7 and CD28 at a molecular level that develops an antagonistic homolog of CTLA-4 and also known to be T-cell antigen receptor. CD28 homolog exhibits higher affinity towards T cells upon combining with B7, allowing it to outcompete CD28 activity and escape the other signals to make a communication with the other T cells [10] (Figure 4.1).

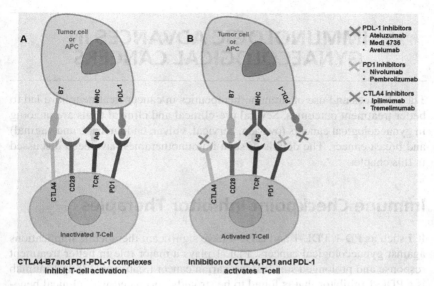

FIGURE 4.1 Mechanism of action of immune checkpoint inhibitors. (A) Antigen-presenting cells (APCs) present antigen via major histocompatibility complex (MHC) and T-cell receptor (TCR) representing the primary signal for activating the T cell. Also, costimulatory signal involving interaction between B7 on APCs and CD28 on T cells are needed to complete T-cell activation and expansion. Different co-receptors function as negative regulators of the immune response at a variety of molecular checkpoints. CTLA-4 expression is raised in T cells during their initial response to antigen. CTLA-4 is delivered to the cell surface in proportion to antigen stimulation and it binds to B7 with a higher affinity than CD28, resulting in T-cell inactivation. PD-1/PD1-L1 regulate inflammatory responses in tissues sustained by effector T cells. Activated T cells upregulate PD-1 and inflammatory signals in the tissue which induce the expression of PD1-L1s and downregulate the activity of T cells. (B) Inhibitors of these particular immune checkpoints block them and increase the T-cell activation and proliferation, resulting in an anti-tumour response.

With promising pre-clinical and clinical findings, adoption and knowledge of immunotherapy in gynaecologic malignancies, including breast cancer, are crucial for better treatment outcomes [11].

Currently, no full-fledged immunotherapeutic treatment options are available against these cancers apart from conventional systemic therapies, including chemo, radio and targeted therapies [12]. In this chapter, we will discuss the utility/advances of immunotherapy in gynaecological cancers including breast cancer.

IMMUNOLOGIC ADVANCES IN GYNAECOLOGICAL CANCERS

The advances and use of immunotherapeutics in cancer treatment have led to better treatment outcomes. Several pre-clinical and clinical trials are ongoing in gynaecological cancers (ovarian, cervical, vulvar, endometrial, and vaginal) and breast cancer. The details of such immunotherapies have been discussed in this chapter.

Immune Checkpoint Inhibitor Therapies

ICI such as PD-1, PDL-1 and CTL-4 have significant therapeutic implications against gynaecological cancers. PDL-1 plays a major role in better treatment response and prolonged survival in ovarian cancer treatment [13]. Ipilimumab is a PDL-1 inhibitor that is found to be strongly correlated with clinical benefits in terms of prolonged survival among ovarian cancer patients [14]. A study showed that US Food and Drug Administration (FDA)-approved pembrolizumab (Keytruda, Merck), a PD-1 inhibitor, along with chemotherapy has proven to be highly effective against cervical cancer [15]. This drug has also been approved for all advanced cancer patients, including gynaecological cancers [16]. A study on lenvatinib plus pembrolizumab showed an overall high survival rate in patients with advanced endometrial cancer stages, where they observed 84% of the patients to be with decreased lesions [17]. In vaginal cancer, a report observed a stabilized outcome in the patients with no deaths on treating with nivolumab [18]. Several clinical trials are ongoing, while few approved immunotherapeutic drugs are available (Table 4.1).

Combination Strategies With PARPi

Poly-(ADP-ribose) polymerase inhibitors (PARPi) are known to be the first and one of the best immunotherapeutic agents for gynaecological cancers, especially ovarian cancer [19]. They are crucial molecules that play a significant role in the repair of DNA single-strand breaks. During cancer, cells that have BRCA1/2 mutation undergo synthetic lethality due to the inhibition of PARP using various FDA-approved drugs such as bevacizumab (Avastin, Genentech Inc., California) [20]. A recent study in BRCA1/2-mutated ovarian cancer patients observed a reduced hazard ratio (between 0.2 and 0.4) of

TABLE 4.1 List of approved immunotherapies in gynaecological and breast cancer.

S.NO.	IMMUNOTHERAPY	BRAND NAME	COMPANY	NATURE	CANCER	TARGET/PATHWAYS
1.	Bevacizumab	Avastin	Roche, Switzerland	Monoclonal antibody	Ovarian cancer	VEGF/VEGFR pathway and inhibits tumour blood vessel growth
2.	Dostarlimab	Jemperli	Glaxo Smith Kline, UK	Checkpoint inhibitor	Ovarian cancer, endometrial cancer, breast cancer	PD-1/PD-L1 pathway
3.	Pembrolizumab	Keytruda	Merck & Co., United States	Checkpoint inhibitor	Ovarian cancer, endometrial cancer, breast cancer, cervical cancer, vaginal cancer	PD-1/PD-L1 pathway
4.	Cervarix	Cervarix	Glaxo Smith Kline, UK	Bivalent vaccine	Cervical cancer	HPV 16/18
5.	Gardasil	Gardasil	Merck Sharp & Dohme Corp., United States	Quadrivalent vaccine	Cervical cancer, vulvar cancer	HPV 6/11/16/18
6.	Gardasil 9	Gardasil 9	Merck Sharp & Dohme Corp., United States	Nine-valent vaccine	Cervical cancer, vulvar cancer, Endometrial cancer, vaginal cancer	HPV6/11/16/18/31/33/45/52/58

(Continued)

TABLE 4.1 (Continued)

S.NO.	IMMUNOTHERAPY	BRAND NAME	COMPANY	NATURE	CANCER	TARGET/PATHWAYS
7.	Margetuximab-cmkb	Margenza	MacroGenics Inc., United States	Monoclonal antibody	Breast cancer	HER2 pathway
8.	Pertuzumab	Perjeta	Genentech, United States	Monoclonal antibody	Breast cancer	HER2 pathway
9.	Sacituzumab govitecan	Trodelvy	Gilead Sciences, United States	Antibody-drug conjugate	Breast cancer	TROP-2 pathway
10.	Trastuzumab	Herceptin	Genentech, United States	Monoclonal antibody	Breast cancer	HER2 pathway
11.	Trastuzumab deruxtecan	Enhertu	AstraZeneca and Daiichi Sankyo Co. Ltd., Japan	Antibody-drug conjugate	Breast cancer	HER2 pathway
12.	Trastuzumab emtansine	Kadcyla	Genentech, United States	Antibody-drug conjugate	Breast cancer	HER2 pathway
13.	Olaparib	Lynparza	AstraZeneca, England	PARP-inhibitor	Ovarian cancer	PARP inhibitor

VEGF, vascular endothelial growth factor; VEGFR, vascular endothelial growth factor receptor; PD-1, programmed cell death protein 1; PDL-1, programmed death-ligand 1; HPV, human papillomavirus; HER2, human epidermal growth factor receptor 2; TROP-2, trophoblast antigen 2.

Source: https://clinicaltrials.gov/.

progression after PARPi treatment [21]. However, its application is limited due to its toxicity profiles [22].

Current Updates on Vaccination Against Gynaecological Cancer

The three prophylactic vaccines against uterine cervix cancer are commercially available in the market: Cervarix (GlaxoSmithKline, UK), Gardasil 9 (Merck Sharp & Dohme Corp.), and Gardasil (Merck & Co., Inc.) (Table 4.1) [23]. These vaccines are targeted against HR-HPV subtypes, as HPV is shown to be one of the most contributing risk factors for cervical cancer [24]. Several trials for the development of therapeutic vaccines are listed in Table 4.2.

TABLE 4.2   List of some vaccines under clinical trials in cervical cancer.

S.NO.	NAME OF THE VACCINE	TARGET	CLINICAL PHASE	OUTCOMES
Therapeutic Vaccine: Live Vector-Based Vaccine				
1.	Live *Listeria monocytogenes* (Lovaxin C)	HPV 16	Completed	No adverse effects, effective in pre-treated metastatic cancer patients, T cell response was observed.
2.	Recombinant vaccinia virus (TA-HPV)	HPV 16 HPV 18	Completed	No clinical side effects were seen, and HPV-specific cytotoxic T cells response has been observed.
3.	Recombinant vaccinia virus (MVA-HPV-IL-2; TG4001)	HPV 16	Phase III	HPV-specific CTLs response to be observed, no clinical side effects have been observed.
4.	*Salmonella enterica serovar typhi* Ty21a	HPV 16	Pre-clinical	Unique in inducing HPV16-neutralizing antibodies in serum and genital secretions
5.	Attenuated *Listeria monocytogenes* (*L. monocytogenes*, LM)	HPV 16	Pre-clinical	Anti-tumour effects, capability to induce CD8+ and CD4+ T cells.

(Continued)

TABLE 4.2 (Continued)

S.NO.	NAME OF THE VACCINE	TARGET	CLINICAL PHASE	OUTCOMES
Therapeutic Vaccine: Bacterial Vector-Based Vaccine				
6.	Recombinant vaccinia virus-based vaccine, modified virus Ankara (MVA)	HPV 16 HPV 18	Phase II	Formation of CD8+ and CD4+ T cells, high level of CTL activity was observed
7.	Lactobacillus family of bacteria	HPV 16 HPV 18	NA	Induce apoptosis, inhibit cell migration and proliferation
8.	Modifies lactic acid bacteria (LAB)	HPV 16	Phase I	Enhanced mucosal immunogenicity against HPV
Therapeutic Vaccine: Peptide Vaccine				
9.	ISA101/ISA101b	HPV 16	Phases I and II	Anti-tumour efficacy was assesses up to one year, HPV-specific immune response was observed.
10.	ISA101b	HPV 16	Phase II	ORR, DOR was assessed up to 3 years
11.	E712–20 and E786–93 peptides linked to the PADRE helper peptide bound to a lipid radical adjuvant: IFA	HPV 16	Phase I	E7-specific CTL response was observed
Therapeutic Vaccine: Protein-Based Vaccine				
12.	SA-4–1BBL	HPV 16	Pre-clinical	Efficacy of the vaccine was associated with robust primary and memory CD4+ and CD8+ T cell responses, Th1 cytokine response, infiltration of CD4+ and CD8+ T cells into the tumour, and enhanced NK cell killing.

S.NO.	NAME OF THE VACCINE	TARGET	CLINICAL PHASE	OUTCOMES
13.	Liposome-polycation-DNA (LPD) particle	HPV 16	Pre-clinical	Robust immune response was observed against HPV.
14.	Fusion protein containing HPV-16 E6 and E7 Adjuvant: ISCOMATRIX [78]	HPV 16	Phase I	Specific CTL response have been observed.
15.	Fusion protein containing HPV-16 L2, E6 and E7 (TA-CIN)	HPV 17	Phase I	E6 and E7-specific CTL responses was assessed.

Therapeutic Vaccine: DNA Vaccine

16.	ZYC101: Zycos 101 plasmid DNA encoding several HLA-A2 epitopes from HPV-16 E7 Encapsulated in microparticles of biodegradable polymer	HPV 16	Phase I	Enhanced response to E7 epitope of HPV
17.	ZYC101	HPV 16 HPV 18	Phase I	HPV-specific CTL response was observed to be induced
18.	INO-3112 DNA Vaccine	HPV 16 HPV 18	Phases I and II	HPV-specific antibody was observed, E6/E7 antigen–specific anti-HPV-16/18 antibody

CTL, cytotoxic T-lymphocytes; HPV, human papillomavirus; DNA, deoxyribonucleic acid; NK, natural killer cells; RNA, ribonucleic acid.
Source: https://clinicaltrials.gov/.

IMMUNOLOGIC ADVANCES IN BREAST CANCER

Breast malignancies are immunoregulatory in nature, and individuals with more immunogenic tumours have a better prognosis. As a result, personalized immunotherapy is becoming an increasingly appealing prospect for treating breast cancer [6].

Breast Cancer Immune Checkpoint Therapies

It has been observed that multiple antibodies inhibit immunological checkpoints which exhibit significant and promising outcomes against breast cancer treatment [25]. Despite the advancement in research, immune checkpoint treatments targeting the CTLA-4, PD-1, PDL-1 and lymphocyte activation gene-3 (LAG-3) pathways are still in clinical trials for breast cancer [26].

The FDA has approved two drugs (nivolumab and pembrolizumab) against the PD-1, which has shown satisfactory overall survival rate and progression-free survival of the patient [27]. One of the most common PD-L1 inhibitors, atezolizumab (MPDL3280A), is now under trial and currently being tested in pre-treated metastatic and PDL-1-positive triple-negative breast cancer patients, where it has shown promising effects [28–29].

LAG3 is another potent immunotherapeutic target found on the activated immune cells, especially on NK cells and T-cell lines [30]. LAG3 possesses a higher affinity than CD4 and is shown to be the probable receptor for MHC class II molecules. LAG-3 is claimed to inhibit various cellular processes like homeostasis of T cells, their proliferation and activation and is also known to contribute significantly towards the suppression behaviour of Tregs. A study on the soluble version of LAG-3 IMP321 suggested that no significant adverse events were found to be associated, and it can be used as a future treatment for breast cancer [31]. Till now, no LAG-3–based approved drugs are available in the market, but several clinical trials to ICI are ongoing.

Monoclonal Antibody (mAb)-Targeted Therapies

For breast cancer, two FDA-approved mAb are available in the market. Trastuzumab (Herceptin, Genentech Inc., California) was the first anti-HER2 mAb to receive FDA approval in 1998, and it remains a critical component of therapy for HER2+ breast cancer. It is directed against the extracellular HER2 domain that inhibits the homodimerization of HER2/neu, hence impairing proliferation, DNA repair, and angiogenesis [5].

Pertuzumab (Perjeta, Genentech, Switzerland), is another approved humanized recombinant mAb, which inhibits HER2/HER3 heterodimerization by interfering with the ligand-dependent HER3 signalling pathway, hence reducing proliferation [10]. The antibody-dependent cell-mediated cytotoxicity reaction induced by pertuzumab leads to the binding of HER2 at a different extracellular domain than the trastuzumab [12]. The combination of trastuzumab, pertuzumab and docetaxel as the first-line treatment was approved by FDA for HER2+ metastatic breast cancer in 2012 [11].

Bispecific Antibodies (bsAb) Therapies

Bispecific antibodies have two arms: one binds with tumour-associated antigen and another with the activator receptor on effector cells, which activates the cytolytic activity for killing the tumour cell [32–33]. In 2009, the first bsAb, named catumaxomab (trifunctional antibody), was approved and targets epithelial cell adhesion molecules in tumours. Blinatumomab was the second approved bsAb and got an official license in 2014 [34]. These antibody-based therapeutics have recently got attention in treating TNBC patients who are highly metastatic and have poor prognosis [35].

CONCLUSION

Immunotherapy has achieved considerable success in exploring and establishing ICI in various cancers. The two most well-known kinds of ICI used in cancer are those that block CTLA-4 and PD-1 ligands. These inhibitors have a number of advantages, including commercial availability, increased survival time, strong vigour, and potency in treatment against cancer cells. Despite achieving great success, the scenario is still not very clear in gynaecological tumours. Although studies have highlighted the importance of checkpoint inhibitors alone or in combination with chemotherapy, VEGF, and PARP inhibitors, still there are some grey areas that needs to be addressed for effective treatment response with improved quality of life post-treatment.

Certainly, immunotherapeutics have the potential to replace conventional cancer treatment. But significant hurdles for cancer ICI are bio-availability, cost-effective and being consistently successful in a broad range of individuals and cancer types with minimum immune-related adverse events [36]. Immunotherapeutics is continuously evolving and is likely to establish its mark significantly in cancer treatments with improved efficacy and minimal side effects in the coming years. To achieve this, research should unravel more tumour antigens which could be defined as immunotherapeutic targets in the future.

REFERENCES

1. Sung H, Ferlay J, Siegel RL, et al. Global cancer statistics 2020: GLOBOCAN estimates of incidence and mortality worldwide for 36 cancers in 185 countries. *CA: A Cancer Journal for Clinicians.* 2021 5;71(3):209–249, doi:10.3322/caac.21660.
2. Funston G, O'Flynn H, Ryan NAJ, et al. Recognizing gynecological cancer in primary care: Risk factors, red flags, and referrals. *Advances in Therapy.* 2018;35(4):577–589, doi:10.1007/s12325-018-0683-3.
3. Beesley VL, Alemayehu C, Webb PM. A systematic literature review of the prevalence of and risk factors for supportive care needs among women with gynaecological cancer and their caregivers. *Supportive Care in Cancer.* 2018/03/01;26(3):701–710, doi:10.1007/s00520-017-3971-6.
4. Hang D, Jia M, Ma H, et al. Independent prognostic role of human papillomavirus genotype in cervical cancer. *BMC Infectious Diseases.* 2017;17(1):391–391, doi:10.1186/s12879-017-2465-y.
5. Burnet M. Cancer: A biological approach. III. Viruses associated with neoplastic conditions. IV. Practical applications. *British Medical Journal.* 1957;1(5023):841–847, doi:10.1136/bmj.1.5023.841.
6. Bondhopadhyay B, Sisodiya S, Chikara A, et al. Cancer immunotherapy: A promising dawn in cancer research. *American Journal of Blood Research.* 2020;10(6):375–385.
7. Le Saux O, Ray-Coquard I, Labidi-Galy SI. Challenges for immunotherapy for the treatment of platinum resistant ovarian cancer. *Seminars in Cancer Biology.* 2020/09/12/, https://doi.org/10.1016/j.semcancer.2020.08.017.
8. Demircan NC, Boussios S, Tasci T, et al. Current and future immunotherapy approaches in ovarian cancer. *Annals of Translational Medicine.* 2020;8(24):1714.
9. Leach Dana R, Krummel Matthew F, Allison James P. Enhancement of antitumor immunity by CTLA-4 blockade. *Science.* 1996/03/22;271(5256):1734–1736, doi:10.1126/science.271.5256.1734.
10. Linsley PS, Greene JL, Brady W, et al. Human B7–1 (CD80) and B7–2 (CD86) bind with similar avidities but distinct kinetics to CD28 and CTLA-4 receptors. *Immunity.* 1994;1(9):793–801, doi:10.1016/S1074-7613(94)80021-9.
11. Dunn GP, Old LJ, Schreiber RD. The three es of cancer immunoediting. *Annual Review of Immunology.* 2004/04/01;22(1):329–360, doi:10.1146/annurev.immunol.22.012703.104803.
12. Mauricio D, Zeybek B, Tymon-Rosario J, et al. Immunotherapy in cervical cancer. *Current Oncology Reports.* 2021/04/14;23(6):61, doi:10.1007/s11912-021-01052-8.
13. Borella F, Ghisoni E, Giannone G, et al. Immune checkpoint inhibitors in epithelial ovarian cancer: An overview on efficacy and future perspectives. *Diagnostics (Basel).* 2020;10(3):146, doi:10.3390/diagnostics10030146.
14. Waldman AD, Fritz JM, Lenardo MJ. A guide to cancer immunotherapy: From T cell basic science to clinical practice. *Nature Reviews Immunology.* 2020/11/01;20(11):651–668, doi:10.1038/s41577-020-0306-5.

15. Wang Y, Li G. PD-1/PD-L1 blockade in cervical cancer: Current studies and perspectives. *Frontiers of Medicine.* 2019/08/01;13(4):438–450, doi:10.1007/s11684-018-0674-4.

16. Charo LM, Plaxe SC. Recent advances in endometrial cancer: A review of key clinical trials from 2015 to 2019. *F1000Research.* 2019;8:F1000 Faculty Rev-849, doi:10.12688/f1000research.17408.1.

17. Makker V, Taylor MH, Aghajanian C, et al. Lenvatinib plus pembrolizumab in patients with advanced endometrial cancer. *Journal of Clinical Oncology: Official Journal of the American Society of Clinical Oncology.* 2020;38(26):2981–2992, doi:10.1200/JCO.19.02627.

18. Naumann RW, Hollebecque A, Meyer T, et al. Safety and efficacy of nivolumab monotherapy in recurrent or metastatic cervical, vaginal, or vulvar carcinoma: Results from the phase I/II checkMate 358 trial. *Journal of Clinical Oncology.* 2019/11/01;37(31):2825–2834, doi:10.1200/JCO.19.00739.

19. Boussios S, Karihtala P, Moschetta M, et al. Combined strategies with poly (ADP-Ribose) polymerase (PARP) inhibitors for the treatment of ovarian cancer: A literature review. *Diagnostics (Basel).* 2019;9(3):87, doi:10.3390/diagnostics9030087.

20. Jiang X, Li X, Li W, et al. PARP inhibitors in ovarian cancer: Sensitivity prediction and resistance mechanisms. *Journal of Cellular and Molecular Medicine.* 2019;23(4):2303–2313, doi:10.1111/jcmm.14133.

21. Tang YH, Lin CY, Lai CH. Development of new cancer treatment by identifying and focusing the genetic mutations or altered expression in gynecologic cancers. *Genes (Basel).* 2021/10/9;12(10), doi:1593 [pii]10.3390/genes12101593.

22. Jesus M, Morgado M, Duarte AP. PARP inhibitors: Clinical relevance and the role of multidisciplinary cancer teams on drug safety. *Expert Opinion on Drug Safety.* 2021/10/20, doi:10.1080/14740338.2022.1996561.

23. Wang R, Pan W, Jin L, et al. Human papillomavirus vaccine against cervical cancer: Opportunity and challenge. *Cancer Letters.* 2020/02/28/;471:88–102, https://doi.org/10.1016/j.canlet.2019.11.039.

24. Das BC, Hussain S, Nasare V, et al. Prospects and prejudices of human papillomavirus vaccines in India. *Vaccine.* 2008/05/23/;26(22):2669–2679, https://doi.org/10.1016/j.vaccine.2008.03.056

25. Gibson J. Anti-PD-L1 for metastatic triple-negative breast cancer. *The Lancet Oncology.* 2015;16(6):e264, doi:10.1016/S1470-2045(15)70208-1.

26. Jain KK. Personalized immuno-oncology. *Medical Principles and Practice.* 2021;30(1):1–16, doi:10.1159/000511107.

27. Nanda R, Chow LQM, Dees EC, et al. Pembrolizumab in patients with advanced triple-negative breast cancer: Phase Ib KEYNOTE-012 study. *Journal of Clinical Oncology: Official Journal of the American Society of Clinical Oncology.* 2016;34(21):2460–2467, doi:10.1200/JCO.2015.64.8931.

28. Emens LA, Braiteh FS, Cassier P, et al. Abstract PD1-6: Inhibition of PD-L1 by MPDL3280A leads to clinical activity in patients with metastatic triple-negative breast cancer. *Cancer Research.* 2015;75(9 Supplement):PD1-6, doi:10.1158/1538-7445.SABCS14-PD1-6.

29. Cimino-Mathews A, Foote JB, Emens LA. Immune targeting in breast cancer. *Oncology.* 2015/05/:375.

30. Triebel F, Jitsukawa S, Baixeras E, et al. LAG-3, a novel lymphocyte activation gene closely related to CD4. *Journal of Experimental Medicine.* 1990;171(5):1393–1405, doi:10.1084/jem.171.5.1393.
31. Brignone C, Gutierrez M, Mefti F, et al. First-line chemoimmunotherapy in metastatic breast carcinoma: Combination of paclitaxel and IMP321 (LAG-3Ig) enhances immune responses and antitumor activity. *Journal of Translational Medicine.* 2010;8:71–71, doi:10.1186/1479-5876-8-71.
32. Chames P, Baty D. Bispecific antibodies for cancer therapy: The light at the end of the tunnel? mAbs. 2009 10–12;1(6):539–547, doi:10.4161/mabs.1.6.10015.
33. Blanco B, Domínguez-Alonso C, Alvarez-Vallina L. Bispecific immunomodulatory antibodies for cancer immunotherapy. *Clinical Cancer Research.* 2021;27(20):5457, doi:10.1158/1078-0432.CCR-20-3770.
34. Buie LW, Pecoraro JJ, Horvat TZ, et al. Blinatumomab: A first-in-class bispecific T-cell engager for precursor B-Cell acute lymphoblastic leukemia. *Annals of Pharmacotherapy.* 2015/09/01;49(9):1057–1067, doi:10.1177/1060028015588555.
35. Dees S, Ganesan R, Singh S, et al. Bispecific antibodies for triple negative breast cancer. *Trends Cancer.* 2021 2;7(2):162–173, doi:S2405–8033(20)30260–0 [pii] 10.1016/j.trecan.2020.09.004.
36. Kalinich M, Murphy W, Wongvibulsin S, et al. Prediction of severe immune-related adverse events requiring hospital admission in patients on immune checkpoint inhibitors: Study of a population level insurance claims database from the USA. *Journal for ImmunoTherapy of Cancer.* 2021;9(3):e001935, doi:10.1136/jitc-2020-001935.

Computational Drug Discovery and Development Along With Their Applications in the Treatment of Women-Associated Cancers

5

Rahul Kumar, Rakesh Kumar,
Harsh Goel, Somorjit Singh
Ningombam and Pranay Tanwar

Contents

DOI: 10.1201/9781003260172-5

INTRODUCTION

Cancer has become a serious life-threatening disease and accounts for relatively 10 million deaths worldwide in 2020 [1]. As of yet, there are about 277 types of cancer, and some cancers, such as those of the breast and ovary, are more gender specific [2]. Globally, the increasing incidence and mortality of cancer pose a major health challenge and have attracted the attention of scientific communities towards the advancement of effective drugs with minimal side effects against cancer.

Drug development is an extensive process of bringing pharmaceutical active compounds from lab to market and costs more than a billion dollars [3]. In the past few decades, CADD has gained popularity after the success-ful deliver of the antiviral drug nelfinavir mesylate against HIV protease and anticancer drugs such as axitinib against VEGF kinase domain and crizotinib against c-MET amplification [4–6]. To counter the duration and cost in the journey of drug development, CADD emerges as an effective approach with an overall aim to escalate the development process of drug for clinical testing. CADD is divided into two based on the different methodologies adopted as SBDD and LBDD (Figure 5.1). In this chapter, we have discussed about the strategies involve in the process of target discovery and different approaches in drug development along with their challenges.

STRUCTURE-BASED DRUG DESIGN

SBDD is a computational approach of predicting the binding pocket within the 3D structure of biological target and optimization of a ligand with considerable binding affinity as well as efficacy.

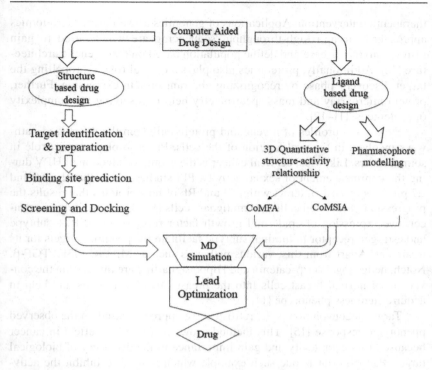

FIGURE 5.1 Detailed pipeline involved in the CADD process. Two different methodologies are widely adopted for computer-aided drug designing. In SBDD, the 3D structure of the target is required followed by the active site prediction and based on these ligands are designed. While in LBDD, only prior knowledge about ligands is required, and designing of the drug will proceed by establishing the ligand 3D quantity structure-activity relationship and pharmacophore modelling. The best-scored ligands are refined through molecular dynamics simulation to find the most promising drug candidate.

Target Prediction

A promising therapeutics target acts as a cornerstone in the process of target-based screening, and it could be either nucleic acid or a protein of different classes [7]. Over the past decades, the development of omics and its application have fostered the discovery of various disease-associated biomarkers [8–9]. Recently, a large number of potential molecular targets for cancer have been reported that can be explore for therapeutic action. There are generally two strategies involve in the identification process: (1) target discovery and (2) target deconvolution. Earlier strategies are based on elucidating the mechanism of disease and its related protein that can be used as a molecular target for further therapeutic intervention. Applications of genomics as well as transcriptomics approaches through high-throughput sequencing are widely used to gain insight into the disease and define population based on their genetic architecture [10]. Additionally, proteomics also plays a critical role in propelling the target discovery phase by recognizing aberrant protein expression. Further, protein microarray and mass spectrometry help in resolving the complexity of proteomes. [11–12].

Expression profiles of a gene and protein enlighten the diversified pathways involved in the proliferation of the cells. PPI also play a direct role in some cancers. Likewise, cervical cancer is the acquired infection of HPV during the commencement of sexual activity. PPI studies reveal that the E6 and E7 proteins of virus interact with p53 and Rb of host proteins that results the progression of infected cells into malignant cells [13]. Likewise in breast cancer, overexpression of epidermal growth factor receptor in HER2+ subtype and estrogen receptor in luminal subtype facilitate the potential targets for its treatment. Apart from this, various pathways such as MAPK, PI3K, TGF-β, Notch, hedgehog, Wnt/β-catenin and Hippo signalling are involved in the conversion of normal breast cells into the breast cancer stem cells and help in acquire stemness phenotype [14].

Target deconvolution is the retrospective approach based on the observed phenotypic response [15]. This method shows its promising effect in cancer because of its complexity and gain importance in the discovery of biological target. Panobinostat is one such example which is used to inhibit the activity of HDACs that is involve in the regulation of gene expression. Currently, by harnessing its therapeutic treatment in BC, panobinostat along with other antineoplastic agents and nucleoside metabolic inhibitors ended in a phase 1/2 clinical trial (NCT00632489) [16].

Preparation of Structure

In SBDD, the target acts as a prerequisite material and relies on the 3D structure as the drug is binding to 3D surface of macromolecules. Usually, 3D structures of macromolecules are elucidated by various experimental approaches such as NMR or x-ray crystallography and resolved structures are deposited in PDB database [17–18]. If the 3D structure of target protein is not available, then it can be determined by using computational methods such as homology (or comparative), threading (or fold recognition) and ab initio (de novo) modelling. Several computational tools are available for 3D structure prediction (Table 5.1). Homology modelling depends upon the sequence homologs with known structure of protein which is used as a template for generating 3D structure of target protein [19–20]. If the homologs have a low sequence identity (<25–30), then the model is constructed by using a threading method which relies on the secondary structures of proteins [21]. Another method is ab initio, used to predict the structure of target protein if no template is available [22]. Once the model is anticipated, stereochemical and geometrical properties are assessed to optimize the quality of the 3D structure.

TABLE 5.1. Computational tools and methods involved in CADD.

3D structure modelling tools/servers	
Alpha fold	https://alphafold.ebi.ac.uk/
I-TASSER	https://zhanggroup.org/I-TASSER/
Modeller	https://salilab.org/modeller/
Robetta	https://robetta.bakerlab.org/
SWISS-MODEL	https://swissmodel.expasy.org/
Phyre2	https://www.sbg.bio.ic.ac.uk/phyre2/html/page.cgi?id=index
HHPred	https://toolkit.tuebingen.mpg.de/tools/hhpred
Bhageerath	https://www.scfbio-iitd.res.in/bhageerath/bhageerath_h.jsp
Binding site prediction tools	
BioLiP	https://zhanggroup.org/BioLiP/
CASTp	https://sts.bioengr.uic.edu/castp/
ConCavity	https://compbio.cs.princeton.edu/concavity/
FindSite	https://cssb.biology.gatech.edu/findsite
fPOP	https://pocket.uchicago.edu/fpop/
SiteComp	https://sitecomp.sanchezlab.org
LigASite	https://www.bigre.ulb.ac.be/Users/benoit/LigASite/index.php?home
Metapocket	https://metapocket.eml.org/
PocketQuery	https://pocketquery.csb.pitt.edu/t
Pocketome	https://www.pocketome.org/
SitesBase	https://www.modelling.leeds.ac.uk/sb/
Active site prediction	https://www.scfbio-iitd.res.in/dock/ActiveSite.jsp
Drug databases	
CancerDR	https://crdd.osdd.net/raghava/cancerdr/
ChEMBL	https://www.ebi.ac.uk/chembldb
Drug bank	https://www.drugbank.ca/
Pubchem	https://pubchem.ncbi.nlm.nih.gov/
Therapeutic target database	https://db.idrblab.net/ttd/
ZINC	https://zinc.docking.org/

(Continued)

TABLE 5.1 (Continued)

Docking	
AutoDock	https://autodock.scripps.edu/
DOCK	https://dock.compbio.ucsf.edu/
GOLD	https://www.ccdc.cam.ac.uk/solutions/csd-discovery/Components/Gold/
Glide	https://www.schrodinger.com/products/glide
ParDOCK	https://www.scfbio-iitd.res.in/pardock/
Docking server	https://www.dockingserver.com/web
FLIPDock	https://flipdock.scripps.edu/
Patchdock	https://bioinfo3d.cs.tau.ac.il/PatchDock/
SwissDock	https://www.swissdock.ch/
Achilles blind docking server	https://bio-hpc.ucam.edu/achilles/

Drug likeness properties	
Lipinski Rule of Five	https://www.scfbio-iitd.res.in/software/drugdesign/lipinski.jsp
SwissADME	https://www.swissadme.ch/
DruLiTo	https://www.niper.gov.in/pi_dev_tools/DruLiToWeb/DruLiTo_index.html
admetSAR	https://lmmd.ecust.edu.cn/admetsar2

Molecular dynamics simulation tools	
AMBER	https://ambermd.org/index.php
Desmond	https://www.schrodinger.com/products/desmond
GROMACS	https://www.gromacs.org/
NAMD	https://www.ks.uiuc.edu/Research/namd/
TINKER	https://tinkertools.org/

Binding Site Characterization

The further step is to predict the ligand binding site for which multiple tools can be used (Table 5.1) [23]. Usually, the co-crystal structure of protein along with its inhibitor or substrate determines the key residues and most favourable binding pocket. However, if the co-crystal structure or information about the key residues are not accessible, then the computational method for predicting the binding pocket is employed, which is based on their interaction energies, and energetically favourable sites are finally selected [24–25].

Screening Small Compound Ligand Libraries

Once the binding site is characterized, the next step is to perform VS with the available structure of target and ligand. VS is a computational strategy use to identify the most likely hit compounds by exploring multiple compound databases or customized libraries (Table 5.1) [26–27]. Apart from VS, de novo is another approach that exploits 3D structural information of target to design a new compound that fits within the binding cavity [28]. Top scored compounds were further filtered based on drug likeliness properties discussed in a later section.

Molecular Docking

Docking involves the estimation of ligand conformation as well as posing within the binding pocket based on the algorithms and scoring functions. It includes various noncovalent interactions together with entropy and enthalpy effects [29]. Once the target and ligands were selected, their preparations are accomplished by the addition of charges followed by binding site mapping where ligand can bind. Various tools used for docking as shown in Table 5.1. The resulting hits after docking are subject to discrete pharmacological validation, such as ADMET properties [30].

LIGAND-BASED DRUG DESIGN

LBDD is another popular method for drug designing, which usually works in the absence of 3D structure of a target protein. The known ligand molecules are investigate to understand the structural and physio-chemical properties which can correlate with the desired pharmacological activity. It is based on the assumption of similar property principle; those compounds display identical structures have similar biological responses upon interactions with the target [31]. This method can also predict novel molecular structures with features facilitating the interactions with the target molecule. 3D QSAR and pharmacophore modelling are the most prominent and commonly used methods in LBDD process that can provide insights into the nature of interactions between drug target and the ligand molecule, thus provide a predictive model suitable for lead compound optimization [32–33].

QSAR

QSAR is a computational approach use to predict the activity of a novel molecule by establishing the relationship between the chemical structures of a group of compounds with a distinct chemical or biological process [34–35]. Molecular features based on the 3D structure of compounds may help define the ligand-receptor interactions. The 3D QSAR method includes descriptors that define the 3D characteristics of a molecule to form a QSAR model. Recently, a variety of ligand-based 3D-QSAR methods such as CoMFA and CoMSIA are built for QSAR determination. CoMFA is one of the most extensively applied 3D QSAR methods [36]. CoMSIA is similar to CoMFA but, unlike CoMFA, the molecular field expression of CoMSIA includes hydrophobic and hydrogen-bond donors. CoMSIA additionally estimates the similarity indices rather than interaction energies by analysing each ligand molecule with a common probe [37–38].

Pharmacophore Modelling

General structural characteristics of ligands can be attained utilizing pharmacophore modelling, which can be used to screen the molecules with these characteristics [39]. A pharmacophore model can be formed from a set of well-known ligands. Despite this, data concerning 3D protein structures or protein-ligand complexes coupled with information about active sites can also be utilized to model a pharmacophore. By examining the binding site, a potential interaction between the active compound and the protein can be understood and pharmacophore models can be established from data on target protein structure followed by virtual screening and lead optimization [40].

MOLECULAR DYNAMICS SIMULATION TO FIND PROMISING DRUGS

Ligand binding sites can be predicted either by experimental studies or computational tools. However, binding site prediction tools often provide multiple binding sites, and users face challenges in opting the right active site. To overcome this limitation, MD simulation provides detailed information about their structural dynamics at an atomic level in a realistic time frame (Table 5.1) [41].

MD in association with other methods can be used to calculate the binding energy of top scored docking ligands and help in finding the most promising drug candidate. Based on the binding energies, ligands are preferred for further in vitro and in vivo validations [42].

DRUG LIKELINESS PROPERTIES

A ligand acts as a good drug candidate if it displays drug like proprieties. Drug likeliness properties can be estimated using various computational tools (Table 5.1). Computational prediction of drug likeliness properties of a ligand is helpful in to minimize the failure of drugs during clinical trials. It can be further subdivided into various features.

Physiochemical Characteristics

RO5 given by C. A. Lipinski describes an initial definition of oral drug-likeness property. The lead molecule should be small having a molecular weight ≤500 daltons, so that it can easily diffuse into the membrane while lipophilicity or logP ≤5. H-bond plays a vital role in determining the specificity of drug binding with the target. The total of H donor should be ≤5 whereas H-bond acceptor or sum of nitrogen and oxygen acceptor is ≤10 [43]. RO5 has been further extended by including another variant, such as molar refractivity, which should range from 40 to 130 [44].

The stability of drugs is governed by their shelf life under defined environmental conditions. Higher shelf life equates to its long stability in turn, it cannot degrade or oxidize easily so that it can be available for selective target. Thus, it prevents itself from multiple binding and reduce their side effects as well as toxicity [45]. Solubility is another concern due to the availability of different pH range from 2 in the stomach to 7.4 in blood. Generally, salt formation method is used to increase the solubility of drug in the distinct profile of pH [46]. Besides, it is necessary to administered drug through its right path to maximize its potency. Generally, the oral route was preferred over other route of administrations because of its convenient, affordability and safety. A major challenge in this route of administration is the bioavailability of the drug, which defines the presence of active concentration or constituent of administered drug at the site of biological destination [47].

Pharmacokinetics Characteristics

In addition to its efficacy against the potent target, a lead compound should be compelled with ADMET features [48]. Absorption of the drug candidate depends upon the permeability of various biological membrane that separates the cells from the foreign particles or external environment, whereas distribution banks on the ability to penetrate physiological barriers such as the gastrointestinal or blood-brain barriers to enter into the blood circulation and extracellular fluid of central nervous system, respectively. The CYP in the liver predicts metabolism of the drug and converts it into metabolites. As a consequence, it can be easily absorbed by the blood plasma and subsequently reach to the effector sites and excreted from the body. Furthermore, the drug may become toxic due to presence of reactive metabolites and their nonspecific interactions with other proteins. To avoid the side effects and to limit the exposure of the drug on other cells or tissues, the above-mentioned pharmacokinetics aspects are to be measured [49–50].

CHALLENGES

In spite of all its advantages, there are several challenges associated with various phases of computational drug designing. The main promise is to determine the optimal target for pharmaceutical intervention. Every disease gene may not be an achievable target as well as its expression profile is confined within the transcription stage and does not indicate about its translation stage. In cases where experimental the 3D structure of target is not available or the sequence identity is <20%, then it can be determined through computational approach which is a complex process and defy its accuracy [22]. During virtual screening, compounds are used in their canonical form and neglect some key factors such as ionization, tautomerism, and protonation, which in turn reduce the significant hits [51]. The scoring algorithm used at the time of docking is intricate and fairly complex. It relies on various approximations and is sometimes out of reach [52]. Also, classical computational has the scaling limitations of simulation for larger biomolecule or complex molecular systems. After meeting with all the necessary functions to be eligible for a successful drug candidate, the majority of oncology drugs fail at the time of phase trials due to lack of safety, efficacy, strategy, and operation [53].

CONCLUSIONS

Cancer, particularly breast cancer, is dominated by the resistance of the cells adopted during its progression in order to escape from their apoptosis. This influences poor prognosis instead of the large number of commercially available drugs. Recent advanced technologies in genomics as well as proteomics unravel the mechanism of drug resistance and explore the alternate potent targets. In a recent decade, CADD acts as a prerequisite part in the drug discovery process by harnessing the exiting theories behind the strategy involved in the lead selection such as ligand interactions and binding energy estimation. Here, we present an integrated approach of in silico drug designing in perspective of breast cancer from lead discovery phase, followed by optimization towards an identifying promising drug candidate. Additionally, MD simulation provides deep insight into the dynamics of atoms and molecules involved in receptor-ligand interactions by simulating them in time scales. At the same time, it also computes binding energy of ligand as well as its residence time within the binding site and enhance the accuracy of putative hits identification. Instead of all the continued development, the above-mentioned challenges remain to be improved. Furthermore, hit compounds are supplemented with in vitro and in vivo validations to elucidate the competency of lead compounds in clinical trials.

SUMMARY

- New drugs are continuously required by the healthcare systems to address unmet medical requirements across distinct therapeutic fields.
- Earlier manoeuvrings are based on illustrating the mechanism of disease that can be used as a molecular target for further therapeutic intervention.
- In the past few decades, CADD has revolutionized the pharmaceutical industry, including the initial stages of research from target discovery and validation, right through to the identification of lead or drug compounds.
- Genomics, transcriptomics and proteomics play a crucial role in investigating and discovering the novel molecular target.

- CADD emerges as an effective approach that intensifies the method of discovering new drugs having therapeutic relevance with minimal side effects in cancer and other diseases.

REFERENCES

1. H Sung et al., CA Cancer J. Clin. (2021). DOI: 10.3322/caac.21660.
2. S H Hassanpour et al., J. Cancer Res. Pract. (2017). DOI: 10.1016/j.jcrpr. 2017.07.001.
3. W Cui et al., Front. Pharmacol. (2020). DOI:10.3389/fphar.2020.00733.
4. S W Kaldor et al., J. Med. Chem. (1997). DOI: 10.1021/jm9704098.
5. K L Meadows et al., Cold Spring Harbor Perspect. Med. (2012). DOI: 10.1101/cshperspect.a006577.
6. R Schwab et al., Lung Cancer (2014). DOI: 10.1016/j.lungcan.2013.10.006.
7. I Gashaw et al., Drug Discov. Today. (2011). DOI: 10.1016/j.drudis.2011.09.007.
8. R Kumar et al., J. Biomol. Struct. Dyn. (2020). DOI: 10.1080/07391102.2020.1740789.
9. R Kumar et al., RSC Adv. (2020). DOI: 10.1039/d0ra07786k.
10. R Spreafico et al., Genes (2020). DOI: 10.3390/genes11080942.
11. J C Somody et al., Drug Discov. Today. (2017). DOI: 10.1016/j.drudis.2017.08.004.
12. X Chen et al., Signal Transduct. Target. Ther. (2020). DOI: 10.1038/s41392-020-0186-y.
13. S Beaudenon et al., BMC Biochem. (2008). DOI: 10.1186/1471-2091-9-S1-S4.
14. S Yousefnia et al., Front. Oncol. (2020). DOI: 10.3389/fonc.2020.00452.
15. J Lee et al., Curr. Opin. Chem. Biol. (2013). DOI: 10.1016/j.cbpa.2012.12.022.
16. C R Tate et al., Breast Cancer Res. (2012). DOI: 10.1186/bcr3192.
17. H M Berman et al., Nucleic Acids Res. (2020). DOI: 10.1093/nar/28.1.235.
18. Zhihai Liu et al., Acc. Chem. Res. (2017). DOI: 10.1021/acs.accounts.6b00491.
19. Y Haddad et al., PLoS Comput. Biol. (2020). DOI: 10.1371/journal.pcbi.1007449.
20. G Studer et al., PLoS Comput Biol (2021). DOI: 10.1371/journal.pcbi.1008667.
21. J Peng et al., Proteins (2011). DOI:10.1002/prot.23016.
22. J Lee et al., From Protein Struct Function Bioinform. (2017). DOI 10.1007/978-94-024-1069-3_1.
23. S Kalyaanamoorthy et al., Drug Discov. Today. (2011). DOI: 10.1016/j.drudis.2011.07.006.
24. M Batool et al., Int. J. Mol. Sci. (2019). DOI: 10.3390/ijms20112783.
25. R Kumar et al., Mol. Divers. (2021). DOI: 10.1007/s11030-021-10210-w.
26. E Lionta et al., Curr. Top. Med. Chem. (2014). DOI: 10.2174/1568026614666140929124445.
27. Z Y Yang et al., Brief Bioinform (2021). DOI: 10.1093/bib/bbaa194.
28. P S Kutchukian et al., Expert Opin. Drug Discov. (2010). DOI: 10.1517/17460441.2010.497534.
29. D B Kitchen et al., Nat. Rev. Drug Discov. (2004). DOI: 10.1038/nrd1549.
30. G M Morris et al., Methods Mol. Biol. (2008). DOI: 10.1007/978-1-59745-177-2_19.

31. G H Loew et al., Pharm. Res. (1993). DOI: 10.1023/a:1018977414572.
32. C Acharya et al., Curr. Comput. Aided Drug. Des. (2011). DOI: 10.2174/157340
    911793743547.
33. J S Mason et al., Curr. Pharm. Des. (2001). DOI: 10.2174/1381612013397843.
34. T Scior et al., Curr. Med. Chem. (2009). DOI: 10.2174/092986709789578213.
35. R P Verma et al., Chem. Rev. (2009). DOI: 10.1021/cr0780210.
36. R D Cramer et al., J. Am. Chem. Soc. (1988). DOI: 10.1021/ja00226a005.
37. G Klebe et al., J. Med. Chem. (1994). DOI: 10.1021/jm00050a010.
38. J Zhao et al., J Biomol Struct Dyn (2020). DOI: 10.1080/07391102.2020.1841678.
39. T Langer et al., Curr. Pharm. Des. (2001). DOI: 10.2174/1381612013397861.
40. Y Kurogi et al., Curr. Med. Chem. (2001). DOI: 10.2174/0929867013372481.
41. X Liu et al., Expert. Opin. Drug. Discov. (2018). DOI: 10.1080/17460441.
    2018.1403419.
42. W Yu et al., Methods Mol. Biol. (2017). DOI: 10.1007/978-1-4939-6634-9_5.
43. C A Lipinski., Drug Discov. Today Technol. (2004). DOI: 10.1016/j.
    ddtec.2004.11.007.
44. A K Ghose et al., J. Comb. Chem. (1999). DOI: 10.1021/cc9800071.
45. C J Briscoe et al., Bioanalysis. (2009). DOI: 10.4155/bio.09.20.
46. A T M Serajuddin., Adv. Drug. Deliv. Rev. (2007). DOI: 10.1016/j.addr.
    2007.05.010.
47. M S. Alqahtani et al., Front. Pharmacol. (2021). DOI: 10.3389/fphar.2021.618411.
48. R Kumar et al.,J.Biomol.Struct.Dyn.(2021).DOI:10.1080/07391102.2021.1897681.
49. C M Song et al., Brief. Bioinform. (2009). DOI: 10.1093/bib/bbp023.
50. D Lagorce et al., Sci. Rep. (2017). DOI: 10.1038/srep46277.
51. T T Brink et al., J. Chem. Inf. Model. (2009). DOI: 10.1021/ci800420z.
52. A E CHO et al., J. Comput. Chem. (2005). DOI: 10.1002/jcc.20222.
53. R K. Harrison., Nat. Rev. Drug Discov. (2016). DOI: 10.1038/nrd.2016.184.

Advances in Nanotechnology for Treatment of Women-Specific Cancers

6

Smriti Arora, Ananya Bishnoi, Gunjan Vasant Bonde and Ashish Mathur

Contents

INTRODUCTION

Despite the fact that women-associated cancers are among the most common cancers worldwide, there are no methods for early detection. Nanomedicine,

DOI: 10.1201/9781003260172-6

nanodiagnosis and nanotheranostics are emerging to cater to unmet needs in oncology and more so are being directed towards women-specific cancers [1]. Nanotechnology (the synthesis and manipulation of materials at the nanoscale level to produce products with new properties) appears to be gaining traction. It has a significant influence on the prevention, diagnosis and treatment of several diseases including cancers. Until nanotechnology arrived, the treatment of cancers relied on surgery, radiation and chemotherapy. These methods are also often referred to as methods of passive therapy. These methods suffer from drawbacks like development of resistance and lack of selectivity thereby leading to cytotoxicity [2]. Immunotherapy is a promising approach to treatment of cancers such many drug conjugates; for example, antibody-drug conjugates (ADC) and peptide-drug conjugates (PDCs) have promising efficacy compared to traditional chemotherapy [3]. Nanotechnology relies on various tools to aid in cancer treatment and diagnosis. These nanotechnology tools include liposomes, dendrimers, nanoparticles, carbon nanotubes and quantum dots (Figure 6.1). Nanoparticles (NPs) can be made from both soft (organic, polymeric) and hard materials (inorganic) of sizes between 1 and 10 nm, and anticancer drugs can be loaded in a variety of configurations. NPs offer advantages over traditional therapy of being specifically targeted at tissue at high concentrations, multiple drugs can be attached, delivery of hydrophobic drugs, protection of drug from harsh conditions of stomach, controlled release of drugs and readout of treatment efficacy [4–5]. Nanotechnology has played a major role in several women-specific cancers also. Some women-specific cancers are ovarian cancer and cervical cancer. These cancers arise in sensitive areas of women's body; therefore, treatment becomes challenging.

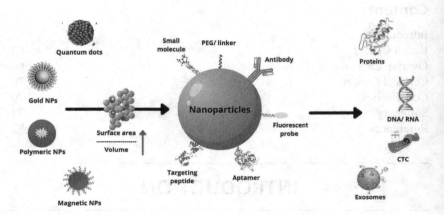

FIGURE 6.1 Types of nanoparticles (NPs) involved in diagnosis, treatment and theranostics of women-associated cancers.

Amongst all, breast cancer (BC) is the most prevalent cancer. In this chapter, women-associated cancers, their diagnosis and treatment using nanotechnology are highlighted. Nanomedicine (nanotechnology used in medicine) has the potential to revolutionize cancer treatments and diagnostics by producing innovative biocompatible nanocomposites for drug delivery [6].

In the following sections, nanotechnology and its application to breast, cervical and ovarian cancers are discussed.

BREAST CANCER

As of January 2021, 3.8 million people were reported with a BC history in the United States (including both women undergoing treatment and finished treatment). It is expected that 30% of newly diagnosed cases in women will be of BC [7–8]. Other gynaecologic malignancies, uterine corpus cancers and ovarian cancers, are estimated to lead to 12,160 and 13,980 deaths in 2019 in the United States, respectively. The major gap that remains in combating this women-associated malignancy is early detection. And even with early diagnosis, 15%–20% patients with stage I disease experience failure [9]. The current treatment of BC involves treatment based on stage of cancer (stages I–III) or metastasis (stage IV). The treatments may be local or systemic. Stages I and II are treated with breast-conserving surgery and radiation therapy. Radiation therapy is known to lead to reduced mortality and relapse. Stage III BC cases are treated with chemotherapy to downsize tumour and breast conservative surgery [10]. If stage III cancer is inflammatory, chemotherapy and mastectomy are recommended. Figure 6.2 illustrates the various stages of BC.

Several clinical-pathological factors discriminate between patients at low (<10%), average (10%–40%) and high risk of relapse. Tumour size, nodal status, tumour grade and age are used to define risk categories. Newer typing methods include HERer2-neu, uPA/PAI-1, gene expression profile and proliferative indices [11]. Stage IV BC is metastatic. In its metastatic situation, BC is incurable but treatable; the main goals are palliative survival and improved quality of life. Other objectives include time to progression, tumour response rate and time to treatment failure. The benefits of adjuvant systemic therapy reducing risk of relapse have been reiterated often [9,11]. Despite this, BC remains a serious public health issue, although the death rates have dropped in recent years, owing to substantially better new therapies for both early-stage illness and those that have demonstrated efficacy in women with advanced disease. NPs offer certain advantages, as they can be functionalized for target specificity and high drug loading [12–13], reduced toxicity and reduced

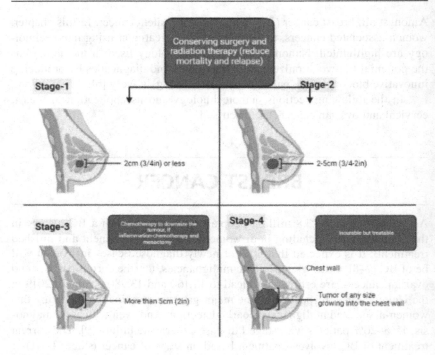

FIGURE 6.2   Various stages of breast cancer.

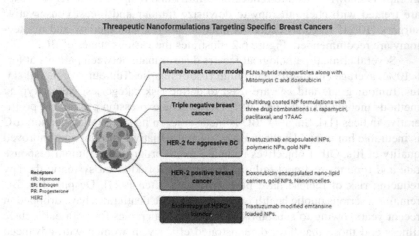

FIGURE 6.3   Advances in nanotechnology that have been successfully used in diagnosis and treatment of HER2-positive breast cancer.

administration frequency [14]. Therapeutic agents of different classes can be combined onto single NP. Furthermore, NPs provide controlled release which normalizes pharmacokinetics, biodistribution and stability of the drugs that independently would give very contrasting pharmacological behaviours [15]. Clearly, NPs have revolutionized diagnosis and therapy of BC. Figure 6.3 summarizes the advances in nanotechnology that have been successfully used in diagnosis and treatment of HER-positive BC.

OVARIAN CANCER

Ovarian cancer (OC) is the fifth-leading cause of death in women, with 313,617 fatalities expected in 2040, as per the predicted data of Globocan's in 2020. The survival rate for OC is 44%, when detected at an early stage. Prognosis is better and survival is much higher in women with timely diagnosis [16]. Unfortunately, due to asymptomatic early tumour stages and late detection, approximately 50%–70% of OC patients relapse, reducing the likelihood of effective therapy [17]. OC patients fall in four categories (Figure 6.4), the first of which are stage I patients with cancer limited to one or two ovaries. Stage II OC extends to pelvic organs (uterus, bladder and fallopian tubes) as well as the ovaries. In stage III, cancer spreads to the abdominal lining, belly, lymph nodes, and other areas, whereas in stage IV it spreads to the lungs, liver, or spleen. Stage IV OC is life-threatening [18]. Epithelial and non-epithelial

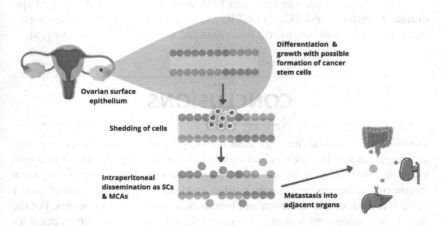

FIGURE 6.4 Various stages of ovarian cancer.

tumours are the two kinds of OCs, with epithelial OC being the most common. The disease's grim statistics show that it is an important and serious issue. There is a need to create new and more intelligent pharmacological treatment techniques to cure this malignancy. The current treatment involves debulking surgery with or without chemotherapy, radiotherapy or a regimen with all three depending on the type and stage of cancer. In OC treatment, several traditional therapies exist like olaprib, bevacizumab, and pazopanib. A variety of drug-loaded NPs can be targeted to tumour cells, resulting in additive and synergistic drug delivery effects. With a view to nanodiagnosis, fluorescently labelled NPs such as QDs, silica or gold NPs and other metal ion–nanoclusters can be used for imaging [19–20]. Biomarkers for OC were found out with the aid of NPs by Castro et al., while Engelberth explored both diagnosis and treatment of OC with the aid of nanoscale devices [21–22].

CERVICAL CANCER

Cervical cancer (CC) is the second most lethal malignancy in women. Despite advancements in therapy, most existing treatments have negative side effects, emphasizing the need for safer and less invasive cervical cancer therapeutic methods. The human papillomavirus (HPV) belongs to the family Papillomaviridae. It is frequently observed in females who are sexually active and causes internal mucosa lesions. There are over 200 HPV serotypes, with HPV 16 and 18 being the present highest risk of cervical cancer.

Several targets such as receptors PI3K/Akt, MAPK, HER2/neu, and epidermal growth factor (EFGR/VEGFR) can be targeted by lipid-based nanoparticles, carbon nanotubes, hybrid nanoparticles, and other formulations [23].

CONCLUSIONS

Development in nanotechnology leads to emerging of various nano-carriers that can target cancer biomarkers and cancer cells selectively enabling more sensitive diagnostics, early identification with minimum tissue sample, long-term monitoring of therapy and tumour burden, and lead to specific necrosis of cancer cells. It provides rapid detection and treatment of uncontrolled tumours. For the time being, using dual stimuli-responsive triggers could be a viable option for increasing tumour selectivity, but more work needs to be done to characterize

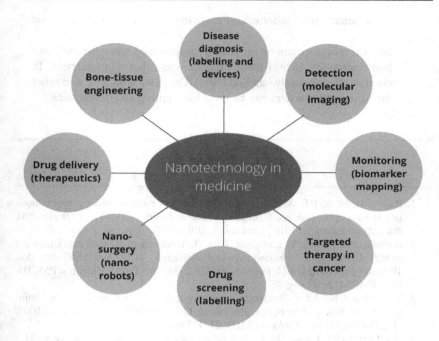

FIGURE 6.5 Key developments in nanotechnology which are evolving at a fast pace to diagnose and treat women-specific cancers.

these systems and improve the scalability of the formulations. Optimized ratiometric loading and compatibility of their efficacy and toxicity profiles are essential considerations for multidrug-carrying nanoparticles. Figure 6.5 illustrates recent developments in nanotechnology which are evolving at a fast pace (some have already evolved) to cater to women-associated cancers.

SUMMARY

- Women-specific cancers, like breast cancer, ovarian cancer, cervical cancer, are more challenging to treat due to their occurrence in more sensitive areas.
- Applications of nanotechnology in cancer treatment not only overcome the pitfalls of conventional therapy but also enable the target-specific controlled drug delivery and monitoring, peptide delivery,

early detection of lesions, and co-delivery of drugs with synergic actions.

- Several receptors can be targeted by lipid-based nanoparticles, carbon nanotubes, hybrid nanoparticles, and other nano-carriers. In contrast, fluorescently labelled NPs, QDs, silica gold NPs, and other metal ion-nanoclusters can be used for imaging and diagnostics.

REFERENCES

1. Rajitha B, Malla RR, Vadde R, et al. Horizons of nanotechnology applications in female specific cancers. *Seminars in Cancer Biology.* 2021 Feb 1;69:376–390. doi: https://doi.org/10.1016/j.semcancer.2019.07.005.
2. Arranja AG, Pathak V, Lammers T, et al. Tumor-targeted nanomedicines for cancer theranostics. *Pharmacological Research.* 2017 Jan;115:87–95. doi: 10.1016/j.phrs.2016.11.014. PubMed PMID: 27865762; PubMed Central PMCID: PMCPMC5412956. eng.
3. Tsuchikama K, An Z. Antibody-drug conjugates: Recent advances in conjugation and linker chemistries. *Protein & Cell.* 2018;9(1):33–46. doi: 10.1007/s13238-016-0323-0. PubMed PMID: 27743348; eng.
4. Farokhzad OC, Langer R. Impact of nanotechnology on drug delivery. *ACS Nano* 2009;3(1):16–20.
5. Bao G, Mitragotri S, Tong S. Multifunctional nanoparticles for drug delivery and molecular imaging. *Annual Review of Biomedical Engineering.* 2013;15:253–82. doi: 10.1146/annurev-bioeng-071812-152409. PubMed PMID: 23642243; PubMed Central PMCID: PMCPMC6186172. eng.
6. Parveen S, Sahoo SK. Polymeric nanoparticles for cancer therapy. *Journal of Drug Targeting.* 2008;16(2):108–123.
7. Howlader N, Noone A, Krapcho M, et al. *SEER Cancer Statistics Review, 1975–2017*, National Cancer Institute. Bethesda, MD. 2020.
8. Liang JW, Idos GE, Hong C, et al. *PanelPRO: A General Framework for Multi-Gene, Multi-Cancer Mendelian Risk Prediction Models. arXiv preprint arXiv:2108.12504.* 2021.
9. Newman LA, Singletary SE. Overview of adjuvant systemic therapy in early stage breast cancer. *The Surgical Clinics of North America.* 2007 Apr;87(2):499–509, xi. doi: 10.1016/j.suc.2007.01.002. PubMed PMID: 17498540; eng.
10. Maughan KL, Lutterbie MA, Ham PS. Treatment of breast cancer. *American Family Physician.* 2010 Jun 1;81(11):1339–1346. PubMed PMID: 20521754; eng.
11. Guarneri V, Conte PF. The curability of breast cancer and the treatment of advanced disease. *European Journal of Nuclear Medicine and Molecular Imaging.* 2004 Jun;31 Suppl 1:S149–161. doi: 10.1007/s00259-004-1538-5. PubMed PMID: 15107948; eng.

12. Bhaskar S, Tian F, Stoeger T, et al. Multifunctional nanocarriers for diagnostics, drug delivery and targeted treatment across blood-brain barrier: Perspectives on tracking and neuroimaging. *Particle and Fibre Toxicology*. 2010 Mar 3;7:3. doi: 10.1186/1743-8977-7-3. PubMed PMID: 20199661; PubMed Central PMCID: PMCPMC2847536. eng.

13. Drbohlavova J, Chomoucka J, Adam V, et al. Nanocarriers for anticancer drugs-new trends in nanomedicine. *Current Drug Metabolism*. 2013 Jun;14(5):547–564. doi: 10.2174/1389200211314050005. PubMed PMID: 23687925; eng.

14. Su H, Wang Y, Gu Y, et al. Potential applications and human biosafety of nanomaterials used in nanomedicine. *Journal of Applied Toxicology: JAT*. 2018 Jan;38(1):3–24. doi: 10.1002/jat.3476. PubMed PMID: 28589558; PubMed Central PMCID: PMCPMC6506719. eng.

15. Ma L, Kohli M, Smith A. Nanoparticles for combination drug therapy. *ACS Nano*. 2013 Nov 26;7(11):9518–25. doi: 10.1021/nn405674m. PubMed PMID: 24274814; PubMed Central PMCID: PMCPMC3894659. eng.

16. Siegel RL, Miller KD, Jemal A. Cancer statistics, 2020. *CA: A Cancer Journal for Clinicians*. 2020 Jan;70(1):7–30. doi: 10.3322/caac.21590. PubMed PMID: 31912902; eng.

17. Rauh-Hain JA, Krivak TC, Del Carmen MG, et al. Ovarian cancer screening and early detection in the general population. *Reviews in Obstetrics & Gynecology*. 2011;4(1):15–21. PubMed PMID: 21629494; PubMed Central PMCID: PMCPMC3100094. eng.

18. Chaurasiya S, Mishra V. Biodegradable nanoparticles as theranostics of ovarian cancer: An overview. *The Journal of Pharmacy and Pharmacology*. 2018 Apr;70(4):435–449. doi: 10.1111/jphp.12860. PubMed PMID: 29380366; eng.

19. Kafshdooz L, Kafshdooz T, Razban Z, et al. The application of gold nanoparticles as a promising therapeutic approach in breast and ovarian cancer. *Artificial Cells, Nanomedicine, and Biotechnology*. 2016 Aug;44(5):1222–7. doi: 10.3109/21691401.2015.1029625. PubMed PMID: 25871281; eng.

20. Pirsaheb M, Mohammadi S, Salimi A, et al. Functionalized fluorescent carbon nanostructures for targeted imaging of cancer cells: A review. *Mikrochimica Acta*. 2019 Mar 8;186(4):231. doi: 10.1007/s00604-019-3338-4. PubMed PMID: 30850906; eng.

21. Castro CM, Im H, Le C, et al. Exploring alternative ovarian cancer biomarkers using innovative nanotechnology strategies. *Cancer and Metastasis Reviews*. 2015 Mar 1;34(1):75–82. doi: 10.1007/s10555-014-9546-9.

22. Engelberth SA, Hempel N, Bergkvist M. Development of nanoscale approaches for ovarian cancer therapeutics and diagnostics. *Critical Reviews in Oncogenesis*. 2014;19(3–4).

23. Zafar A, Alruwaili NK, Imam SS, et al. Novel nanotechnology approaches for diagnosis and therapy of breast, ovarian and cervical cancer in female: A review. *Journal of Drug Delivery Science and Technology*. 2021;61:102198.

Identifying Breast Cancer Treatment Biomarkers Using Transcriptomics

7

Ashfaq Ali Mir

Contents

INTRODUCTION

Cancer is a multigene disorder that could arise from changes in the mutational landscape, transcriptional and epigenetic setup of an individual. Tamoxifen started the trend of precision oncology in breast cancer (Jordan,

1993) Targeted cancer therapy has evolved ever since, and now single genes like BRAF or composite signatures are being used for breast cancer treatment. There is a growing list of FDA-approved targeted cancer therapies that are using gene targets like BRCA1, BRAF, CKIT and EGFR checking for mutations or EGFR and androgen receptors for changes in the expression or checking fusions in NTRK. Microsatellite instability has also been validated as a histology-agnostic biomarker for FDA approval for the likes of entrectinib. There is an ever-growing list for genome-driven therapies following the scale of clinical actionability for molecular targets (ESCAT) of the European Society for Medical Oncology (ESMO). The clinical benefits of such treatments are on the rise.

Multi-cancer detection tests like GRAIL (Klein *et al.*, 2021) using DNA-methylation or comprehensive genome profiling using novel immuno-oncology signatures like tumour mutation burden, microsatellite instability, DNA repair and homologous recombination deficiency (HRD) have been gaining momentum. NGS-based cancer tests and therapies have shown increasing adoption with promising clinical benefits. The future of precision medicine in oncology lies in the adoption of whole genome, exome, transcriptome and epigenome-based tests and combining information from these tests using the multiomics approach to get a complete picture at the multi-dimensional scale.

NGS-BASED APPROVED TESTS AND THEIR LIMITATIONS

FDA has approved many NGS companion diagnostic tests for multiple cancers and biomarkers using liquid biopsies which are non-evasive like Foundation Medicine Inc.'s Liquid CDx test for detecting biomarkers using cell-free DNA isolated from plasma. Approved biomarker indicators include mutational profiling in BRCA1 and BRCA2, which the major known breast cancer risk genes. This test uses 324 gene panels and checks for copy number changes, gene fusions, tumour mutation burden, and changes in PDL-1 (IHC). Rucaparib (RUBRACA, Clovis Oncology, Inc.) is used to treat patients with ovarian cancers using BRCA1 and BRCA2. The PIK3CA gene is used for breast cancer detection with Alpelisib (PIQRAY, Novartis Pharmaceutical Corporation).

However, there are a few limitations due to tumour heterogeneity, static or dynamic, and different sequencing techniques. It is always suggested to have fresh biopsies not older than 7 years, especially for FFPE cancer tissue samples. One of the most frequently seen mutations called "driver mutations" has been puzzling the researchers, which are also present in normal tissue and benign conditions. Therefore, an effort needs to be done to standardize NGS tests on real-world case studies using a larger pool of patients and recording the therapeutic interventions in reports to establish utility based on the FDA criteria.

ABERRANT TRANSCRIPTS AS BIOMARKERS

The receptor tyrosine kinase c-MET gene is a very well-known proto-oncogene that has been found to be involved in multiple cancers including breast cancer. The HGF/c-Met pathway has been shown to be associated with breast cancer. This gene controls many cellular functions important for organ development and cancer progression. A variety of cancers have reported anomalous transcriptional signalling in this gene. Aberrant transcription in this gene has been reported extensively (Miglio *et al.*, 2018). Demethylation of the antisense promoter of the LINE-1 in the second intron of this gene produces antisense transcripts which were found to be enriched in triple-negative breast cancer (TNBC) and high-grade carcinomas. Higher levels of the aberrant transcript have been strongly correlated with aggressive cancers. Interestingly, cell lines expressing the aberrant transcript were initially identified in silico. This highlights the importance of transcriptomics-based analysis using RNA-Seq for proto-oncogene biomarker detection and its usefulness. There are many public resources like euL1db (Mir *et al.*, 2014) (http://eul1db.ircan.org/), which report transposable elements in the human genome and can be useful in understanding the correlation between genome polymorphism and phenotype and disease.

The question that arises now is that is it possible to track aberrant transcripts using NGS sequencing like RNA-Seq. This scenario was studied by Mir (2015), while performing transcriptome assembly of MCF7 cell lines RNA-Seq data. However, it must be noted that to repeat such analysis, the sequencing depth should be pretty high, and transcriptome mappers like STAR (Dobin *et al.*, 2013) or HISAT (Kim *et al.*, 2015), which allow soft clipping, should be used.

Mir (2015), while analysing transcriptome data from MCF breast cancer cell lines, were able to detect aberrant transcripts after performing the transcriptome assembly of RNA-Seq pair-end reads (Figure 7.1). Interestingly, the discordant reads whose one of the mate-pair was unmapped in the genome mapping were mapped to the mobile DNA sequences of LINE-1 retrotransposons

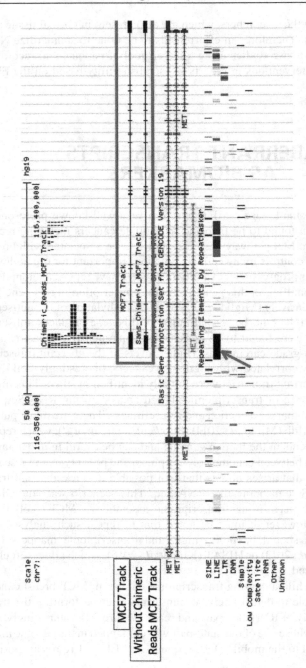

FIGURE 7.1 Transcriptome assembly of MCF cell line which shows aberrant transcripts compared to the reference transcripts from GENCODE in the UCSC Genome Browser. The horizontal box highlights assembled transcripts with or without discordant reads mapping to the LINE-1 transposons for the MET gene. Discordant reads mapping to the LINE-1 have been shown at the top. These reads form the alternative first exon in the second intron of MET gene while disrupting normal transcription.

from the Repeat Masker database (Jurka *et al.*, 2005). Two-tier transcriptome assemblies were performed to check the contribution of discordant reads mapping to the LINE-1 transposon in the second intron of the MET gene in isoform structure. It was observed that when discordant reads labelled as chimeric reads whose one mate mapped to the reference genome and another mate to the mobile element did contribute to the part of the first exon for the aberrant transcript at least in the transcriptome assembly. Conceptually, this transcript is formed by the antisense promoter of the LINE-1, which is activated by the methylation changes in its antisense promoter. In general, it is possible to track methylation changes in the genome by using bisulfite DNA methylation sequencing. Locating differentially methylated regions and looking for consequent changes in the transcriptome might be very useful. In the case of liquid biopsies using cell-free DNA, it might be also possible to add deconvolution analysis for locating the tissue of origin and subsequent cancer specificity analysis using the Genotype-Tissue Expression datasets from the GTEx database (Consortium, 2013). Locating H3K27ac marks using ChIP-Seq histone mark sequencing might help in checking the functional signal for the antisense promoter or promoter in aberrant transcripts. Even simple human-spliced ESTs can help in reinforcing the possibilities.

This clearly shows that transcriptomics along with other omics techniques can help in identifying the aberrant transcripts from cancer samples and check for their functional characteristics. Much has been published about contribution of splicing in detecting cancer-related transcriptional changes (Meng *et al.*, 2019).

SPLICING AND TRANSCRIPTOME-WIDE ASSOCIATION STUDY BIOMARKERS

Splicing can provide clues about overall transcriptional degradation in a sample and can be a great biomarker. For example, a higher proportion of alternate last exons would mean that transcription has been stopped prematurely more often in a cancer sample versus a normal sample comparison scenario. A higher proportion of alternative first exons would highlight higher rates of changes in the protein structure. Figure 7.2 highlights changes in the transcriptome for a control versus a low-grade cancer versus a high-grade cancer. The sample was from RNA-Seq cancerous liquid biopsy.

There are many cases where cancer has been detected by observing the alternate splicing. Androgen receptor preferentially induces transcription from an alternative first exon in TPD52 in prostate cancer (Rubin *et al.*, 2004). Other

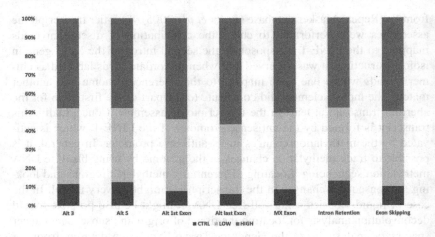

FIGURE 7.2 Changes in the alternative splicing event count percentage using RNA-Seq data between a control versus low-grade versus high-grade cancer samples from the liquid biopsy.

cases like Novel exon that appears to be a novel transcription start site preferentially induced by AR-V7 in PGAP2 known to be induced to a lesser extent by AR (Rana *et al.*, 2021). Similarly, several cases of alternate splicing case have been studied which contribute to breast cancer metastasis (Meng *et al.*, 2019).

Transcriptome-wide association studies (TWAS) have been shown to provide causal genes by integrating the expression quantitative loci with genome-wide association studies. Transcriptome-wide association studies were shown to provide breast cancer risk causal genes by estrogen receptor status (Feng *et al.*, 2020). Some studies were also done to understand the breast cancer outcomes in diverse populations and pinning down the causal genes (Bhattacharya *et al.*, 2020).

TRACKING CANCER CELLS USING NON-EVASIVE LIQUID BIOPSIES

DNA methylation changes can provide excellent biomarkers by checking for differential methylation and using deconvolution for zooming down to cancer cells for practically every cancer type including ovarian and breast cancers. The underlying core methodology for these tests is that blood contains DNA fragments from tumours and other cells (Huang *et al.*, 2019). Since this cell-free DNA is derived from the genome, it can show which of the cells in our body have become carcinogenic.

Recently, there has been a lot of effort in developing NGS-based liquid biopsy-based tests by bisulfite sequencing using cell-free DNA from liquid biopsies like urine and blood. Many companies like GRAIL (Klein *et al.*, 2021) have developed NGS-based multi-cancer detection tests. This can in the future reduce organ-specific screening and make it possible to track and detect cancer even in their early phase. For the GRAIL test, all that is needed is a blood sample tube. GRAIL claims to detect more than 50 cancer types using just one test. Just to set things straight, currently only five cancer types, including breast and cervical cancers, are screened. Therefore, this kind of screening can add a new dimension to cancer screening for other types of cancers in early phase detection.

Multiple computational methods (Scott *et al.*, 2020) have been developed to identify cell-type-specific methylation signals using DNA methylation for whole-genome bisulfite sequencing both from reference-based and non-reference-based. This field is known as immunomethylomics and is part of the collective effort of epigenome-wide association studies (EWAS). Methods that don't need cell sorting have also been developed (Rahmani *et al.*, 2019).

Since DNA methylation changes can enhance DNA damage processes in our genome. Therefore, tracing DNA damage or repair-related pathways in differentially methylated regions with simple analysis like gene set enrichment analysis can provide a bird's-eye view of the carcinogenic gene action or pathways (Subramanian *et al.*, 2005).

USE OF GENOMIC BIOMARKERS IN SYNC WITH TRANSCRIPTOMIC BIOMARKERS

Genomic biomarkers like somatic structural variations (Tubio, 2015) can help in zooming in to the change-maker genes in cancer. Previously studies have shown that structural variations in circadian genes like Per3 can increase the risk of breast cancer (Zhu *et al.*, 2005). Therefore, it's worth looking at structural variations like insertions, deletions, copy number variations, and translocations in trying to understand the links between what is happening in the genome and how it is affecting the transcriptome.

There are public repositories where researchers have tried to understand the links between structural variations in the genome and disease or phenotype like dbGap (Tryka *et al.*, 2013), euL1db (Mir, Philippe and Cristofari, 2014) and ClinVar (Landrum *et al.*, 2018). Data in some of these repositories has been provided at the sample, family, and even population levels. Researchers have also studied the patterns of somatic structural variations in cancer (Li *et al.*, 2020). Things like aberrant transcripts or antisense transcripts, splicing, and fusion genes all these aspects can add up when we try to have a holistic view. How much it is going to help in clinical decision-making is something that only time will tell.

CONCLUSION

Transcriptomics-based biomarkers are adding a new layer of information in the clinical decision-making process for breast, ovarian and other cancer types. This is especially the case with non-evasive liquid biopsies that can make things much easier for patients, reducing risks. In general, NGS-based testing can improve response rate and progression-free survival. Cell-free DNA methylation coupled with transcriptional splicing has provided deeper insights, more biomarkers and causal genes for real-world testing. However, the tissue collection strategy for NGS will still be a matter of debate for some time to come. Costs, privacy and clinical data management will surely be the key areas to look for in the future.

SUMMARY

- NGS-based testing is making faster, reproducible and non-evasive ways of cancer detection possible.
- DNA methylation using whole-genome bisulfite sequencing is helping in screening for a wide range of cancers, including women-related cancers.
- Transcriptomics is helping to identify causal genes contrary to only identifying loci-specific changes in the genome.
- RNA-Seq is helping us in identifying aberrant and antisense transcripts that can act as potent biomarkers for zooming in to the oncogenes.
- Somatic structural variations have shown potential in detecting women-related cancers.
- Tracking splicing changes in the transcripts has added a new dimension in studying the aspects of changes in the genome and their effects on the transcriptome.

REFERENCES

Bhattacharya, A. *et al.* (2020) "A framework for transcriptome-wide association studies in breast cancer in diverse study populations," *Genome Biol*, 21(1), p. 42. doi:10.1186/s13059-020-1942-6.

Consortium, Gte. (2013) "The genotype-tissue expression (GTEx) project," *Nat Genet*, 45(6), pp. 580–585. doi:10.1038/ng.2653.

Dobin, A. *et al.* (2013) "STAR: Ultrafast universal RNA-seq aligner," *Bioinformatics (Oxford, England)*. 2012/10/25, 29(1), pp. 15–21. doi:10.1093/bioinformatics/bts635.

Feng, H. *et al.* (2020) "Transcriptome-wide association study of breast cancer risk by estrogen-receptor status," *Genet Epidemiol*, 44(5), pp. 442–468. doi:10.1002/gepi.22288.

Huang, C.-C., Du, M. and Wang, L. (2019) "Bioinformatics analysis for circulating cell-free DNA in cancer," *Cancers (Basel)*, 11(6). doi:10.3390/cancers11060805.

Jordan, V.C. (1993) "Fourteenth gaddum memorial lecture. A current view of tamoxifen for the treatment and prevention of breast cancer," *Br J Pharmacol*, 110(2), pp. 507–517. doi:10.1111/j.1476-5381.1993.tb13840.x.

Jurka, *et al.* (2005) "Repbase Update, a database of eukaryotic repetitive elements." *Cytogenet Genome Res*. 110(1–4), pp. 462–467. doi:10.1159/000084979.

Kim, D., Langmead, B. and Salzberg, S.L. (2015) "HISAT: A fast spliced aligner with low memory requirements," *Nat Methods*, 12(4), pp. 357–360. doi:10.1038/nmeth.3317.

Klein, E.A. *et al.* (2021) "Clinical validation of a targeted methylation-based multi-cancer early detection test using an independent validation set," *Ann Oncol*, 32(9), pp. 1167–1177. doi:10.1016/j.annonc.2021.05.806.

Landrum, M.J. *et al.* (2018) "ClinVar: Improving access to variant interpretations and supporting evidence," *Nucleic Acids Res*, 46(D1), pp. D1062—D1067. doi:10.1093/nar/gkx1153.

Li, Y. *et al.* (2020) "Patterns of somatic structural variation in human cancer genomes," *Nature*, 578(7793), pp. 112–121. doi:10.1038/s41586-019-1913-9.

Meng, X. *et al.* (2019) "Contribution of alternative splicing to breast cancer metastasis," *J Cancer Metastasis Treat*, 2019/03/22, 5, p. 21. doi:10.20517/2394-4722.2018.96.

Miglio, U. *et al.* (2018) "The expression of LINE1-MET chimeric transcript identifies a subgroup of aggressive breast cancers," *Int J Cancer*, 143(11), pp. 2838–2848. doi:10.1002/ijc.31831.

Mir, A.A. (2015) *Structural variations of the human genome and transcriptome induced by LINE-1 retrotransposons*. Université Nice Sophia Antipolis.

Mir, A.A., Philippe, C. and Cristofari, G. (2014) "euL1db: The European database of L1HS retrotransposon insertions in humans," *Nucleic Acids Res*, 43(Database issue), pp. D43–47. doi:10.1093/nar/gku1043.

Rahmani, E. *et al.* (2019) "Cell-type-specific resolution epigenetics without the need for cell sorting or single-cell biology," *Nat Commun*, 10(1), p. 3417. doi:10.1038/s41467-019-11052-9.

Rana, M. *et al.* (2021) "Androgen receptor and its splice variant, AR-V7, differentially induce mRNA splicing in prostate cancer cells," *Sci Rep*, 11(1), p. 1393. doi:10.1038/s41598-021-81164-0.

Rubin, M.A. *et al.* (2004) "Overexpression, amplification, and androgen regulation of TPD52 in prostate cancer," *Cancer Res*, 64(11), pp. 3814–3822. doi:10.1158/0008-5472.CAN-03-3881.

Scott, C.A. *et al.* (2020) "Identification of cell type-specific methylation signals in bulk whole genome bisulfite sequencing data," *Genome Biol*, 21(1), p. 156. doi:10.1186/s13059-020-02065-5.

Subramanian, A. *et al.* (2005) "Gene set enrichment analysis: A knowledge-based approach for interpreting genome-wide expression profiles," *Proc Natl Acad Sci U S A*, 102(43), pp. 15545–15550. doi:10.1073/pnas.0506580102.

Tryka, K.A. *et al.* (2013) "NCBI's database of genotypes and phenotypes: dbGaP," *Nucleic Acids Res*, 42(Database issue), pp. D975–979. doi:10.1093/nar/gkt1211.

Tubio, J.M.C. (2015) "Somatic structural variation and cancer," *Brief Funct Genomics*, 14(5), pp. 339–351. doi:10.1093/bfgp/elv016.

Zhu, Y. *et al.* (2005) "Period3 structural variation: A circadian biomarker associated with breast cancer in young women," *Cancer Epidemiol Biomarkers Prev*, 14(1), pp. 268–270. Available at: www.ncbi.nlm.nih.gov/pubmed/15668506.

Integrating CADD and Herbal Informatics Approach to Explore Potential Drug Candidates Against HPV E6 Associated With Cervical Cancer

8

Arushi Verma, Jyoti Bala, Navkiran Kaur and Anupama Avasthi

Contents

DOI: 10.1201/9781003260172-8
                                                            85

INTRODUCTION

Cancer is a large group of diseases that can start in almost any organ or tissue of the body when abnormal cells proliferate uncontrollably, transcend their usual boundaries and invade adjacent sections of the body. Cervical cancer is one of the most common cancers at both the national and global levels among women, mostly appearing to be an age-standardized disease, affecting middle-aged women (30–40+ years). One of the prime causes of cervical cancer is human papillomavirus (HPV) infection, accounting for about 83.78% of cases in India [1] and 55% globally [2]. Amongst various viral oncoproteins, E6 plays a vital role in changes of cervical epithelial cells by attacking and blocking the function of p53, also known as TP53 (Tumor Protein 53). Almost 50% of cancer cases are found to be due to p53 mutation/inactivation. E6 protein binds with p53 and E6-AP (E6-associating protein) to form a trimer, which leads to the ubiquitination of TP53. Now, 26S proteasome recognizes ubiquitinated TP53 and degrades it, which leads to virus-induced cellular transformations. Due to such simultaneous degradation of TP53, its adequate level decreases in the body, and it directly affects the apoptosis and DNA repair mechanisms, which leads to increased cell proliferation [3]. Computer-aided drug discovery has two approaches: a structure-based approach and a ligand-based approach. In this project, the structure-based approach has been applied. It utilizes the knowledge of three-dimensional structure of our target (biological) obtained through NMR spectroscopy or x-ray crystallography methods [4] to search candidate drugs that can bind with high affinity and selectivity to it. Today, the majority of treatments available for cervical cancer are quite invasive, with multiple side effects. Herbal informatics allows us to look into the plant domains in search of phytocompounds/ligands having lesser side effects and greater efficacy; once the ligands are proposed in silico, their efficacy can be confirmed in pre-clinical and clinical trials.

METHODS AND MATERIALS

Identification of a therapeutic target and sequence retrieval: Information about cervical cancer and detailed literature search conducted in

NCBI [5] database. The primary sequence of HPV E6 protein was retrieved from Uniprot [6] (ID: P03126) in FASTA format.

Target structure analysis and preparation: Family and domain studies were performed using Uniprot. Protparam [7] to study physical and chemical composition of the protein and secondary structure analysis was done using SOPMA [8]. PSIPRED [9] was used to predict 2D protein structure and nature of individual amino acid. JPred [10] server was used to obtain secondary structure wiring diagram, to give us a realistic idea on 2D structure. Tertiary structure of the protein was obtained from RCSB PDB database (ID: 4GIZ) [11]. The structure originally obtained was edited in UCSF Chimera interface [12]. Pathway analysis of HPV 16 in human body and its interaction was studied using STRING Viruses database [13]. HPV infection analysis from KEGG database [14] informed us about pathways where E6 protein was involved.

Ligand preparation: Identification and analysis done thorough literature search through NCBI indicated Luteolin [15] and Daphnoretin [16] as anti-neoplastic, antiviral agents and apoptosis inducing. Physiochemical analysis were done using PubChem [17] and 3-D structures of both the hits were built and visualized. ChEMBL [18] and Drugbank [19] were used to gather relevant information about the ligands like its sources, alternative forms, activity charts, clinical data and so forth.

Molecular docking: Molecular docking studies were performed using PatchDock server [20] and docking results were visualized using Chimera in 3D and 2D. Docking analysis was performed using Protein-Ligand Interaction Profiler [21].

Drug likeliness prediction: ADME analysis was done using the swissADME [22] tool, and toxicity prediction for both hits was performed on various parameters on the preADMET tool [23]. Bioactivity and molecular activity scores for various properties were obtained from Molinspiration [24].

RESULTS AND DISCUSSION

Computer-aided drug designing can be implemented in two ways, of which we are adopting the structure-based approach, which means we have first identified a particular disease model and after detailed study have selected a target protein, followed by ligand selection. The primary and secondary structure of target protein E6 (Gene E6) of Organism *Human papillomavirus type 16* were obtained from Uniprot (Id: P03126), as depicted in Figure 8.1A and 8.1B. The

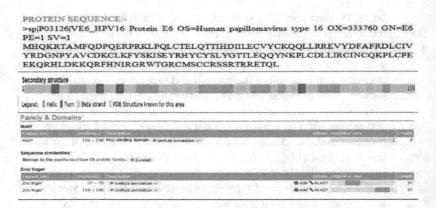

FIGURE 8.1 (A) FASTA sequence of E6 protein; studied in HPV. It consists of 158 amino acids, starting from methionine and ending with leucine. (B) Secondary structure of E6 protein. (C) Family and domain studies of HPV E6 protein, performed on Uniprot.

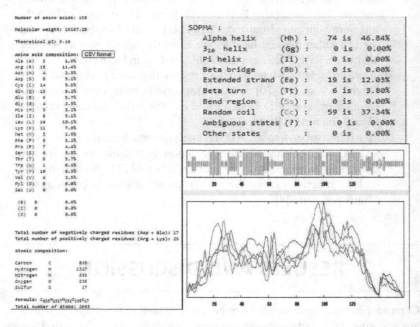

FIGURE 8.2 (A) Amino acid and atomic composition in E6 protein observed in Protparam. (B) Secondary protein structure analysis of E6 protein using SOPMA depicts maximum alpha helices contribution for about 46.84% followed by random coils for 37.34%. (C) Secondary structure prediction of E6 protein using SOPMA.

protein sequence is 158 amino acids long. Its family and domain search reveals the presence of PDZ binding domain or LxxLL binding pocket and two Zn^{2+} finger domains (Figure 8.1C).

The atomic composition and nature of E6 protein were studied (Figure 8.2A), which indicated a significant amount of arginine contribution (11.4%) towards the protein sequence, followed by leucine (10.1%), indicating a greater positive charge overall (Arg + Lys = 29). The theoretical pI came out as 9.16. Secondary structure prediction using SOPMA indicated where maximum of alpha helices, followed by random coils and extended strands (Figure 8.2B, C).

The structural analyses were done using PSIPRED, where various structure components were represented through colours. The results are depicted in Figure 8.3A and 8.3B. The secondary E6 structure as obtained from Jpred indicated the presence of seven helices and their six strands, 12 beta turns, and two beta hairpins, as depicted in Figure 8.3C.

The tertiary structure of protein was obtained from RCSB PDB. It was edited in Chimera to obtain chains C and D of E6 protein from the complex (Figure 8.4). The STRING viruses database included reaction and relationship networks between various human and HPV E6 protein (Figure 8.5A).

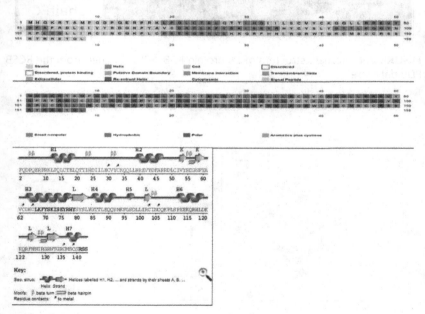

FIGURE 8.3 (A) Structure prediction of E6 oncoprotein in PSIPRED, depicting what kind of structure is executed by which section of amino acids. (B) Nature of different amino acids present in E6 oncoprotein is indicated by varying grey scales, studied in PSIPRED. (C) Secondary structure of 4GIZ observed in Jpred: a wiring diagram of secondary structure.

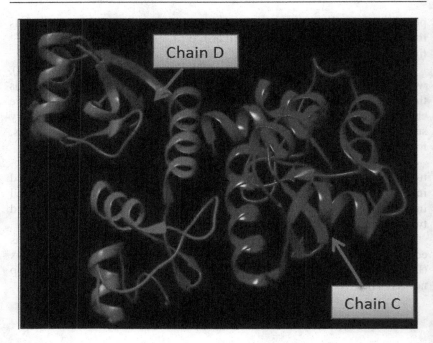

FIGURE 8.4   Tertiary structure of E6 protein PDB 4GIZ obtained from the RCSB PDB database.

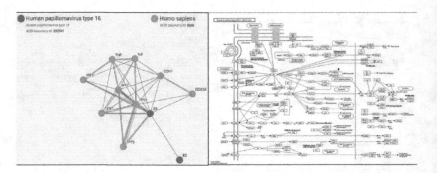

FIGURE 8.5   (A) Pathway analysis STRING pathway of E6 molecular interactions (after the HPV genome interacts with human cells). (B) HPV infection pathway analysis from KEGG database. The role of E6 protein is denoted in different shade throughout.

The KEGG database provides a detailed examination of E6's role in various metabolic reactions in our body. It aids in understanding the molecular dynamics of the disease. All the major E6-associated interactions that occur in the body during HPV infection are depicted in Figure 8.5B. We found its involvement in several metabolic pathways, like the Wnt signalling pathway, inhibition of apoptosis, cellular immortalization, inhibition pathway of host antiviral response and so forth. These all indicated strong E6 involvement in the development of cancer.

For ligand analysis, two probable hits were short-listed after a thorough literature search: luteolin (an anti-cancerous, anti-allergenic, antioxidant, anti-inflammatory agent) [25] and daphnoretin (an anti-apoptotic, anti-cancerous [26], and antiviral (CHEBI: 4324) agent). Physicochemical properties (structure and formula, source, class of compound, molecular weight, SMILES id, H-bond acceptors and donors, topological surface area, etc.) were analysed and are tabulated in Table 8.1. PubChem's SMILES notation was used in Chimera

TABLE 8.1 Potential phytochemical ligands (luteolin and daphnoretin) and their physiochemical property analysis.

PHYTOCHEMICAL PROPERTIES	LUTEOLIN	DAPHNORETIN
Structure		
Source	Salvia tomentosa	Wikstroemia indica
Class	Flavones	Benzopyrans (coumarins)
PubChem ID	5280445	5281406
Mol. Weight	286.24	352.3
Mol. Formula	$C_{15}H_{10}O_6$	$C_{19}H_{12}O_7$
H-Bond Acceptors	6	7
H-Bond Donors	4	1
SMILES Notation	C1=CC(=C(C=C1C2=CC(=O)C3=C(C=C(C=C3O2)O)O)O)O	COC1=C(C=C2C(=C1)C=C(C(=O)O2)OC3=CC4=C(C=C3)C=CC(=O)O4)O
TSA	107 Å²	91.3 Å²
XLogP3	1.4	3.3

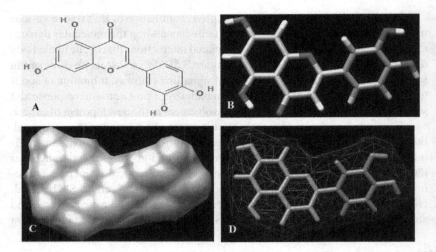

FIGURE 8.6 Chemical structure (secondary and tertiary structure) of luteolin. (A) Secondary structure of luteolin. (B–D): Tertiary structure data collected from PubChem and further built on Chimera. Visualization was done on the same tool as well.

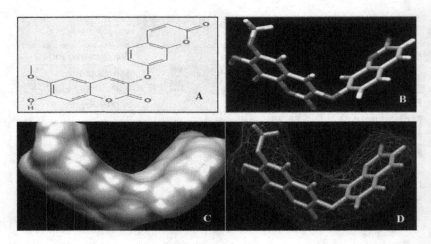

FIGURE 8.7 Chemical structure (secondary and tertiary structure) of daphnoretin. (A) Secondary structure of daphnoretin. (B–D) Tertiary structure data collected from PubChem and further built on Chimera. Visualization was done on the same tool as well.

to create 3D structures of phytochemicals and appropriately processed and viewed on Chimera (Figures 8.6, 8.7).

Results of docking analysis (highest scores) done using PatchDock tool is available in Table 8.2. Visualization and bond analysis were done using Chimera. For better visualization, they were examined in 3D (ribbon) and 2D atom formats, as shown in Figures 8.8A and 8.9A. Molecular docking analysis

TABLE 8.2 Molecular docking results: target HPV E6 protein and luteolin and daphnoretin ligands were docked using PatchDock server.

PATCHDOCK RESULTS		HIGHEST SCORE	
S.No.	Ligand	Score	ACE
1	Luteolin	3312	−140.08
2	Daphnoretin	3844	−158.78

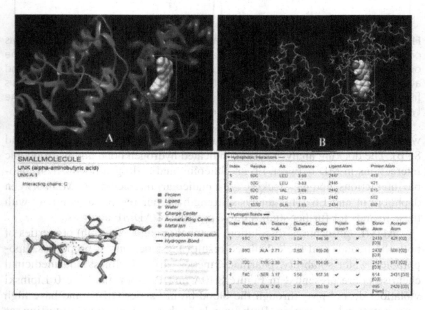

FIGURE 8.8 HPV E6 protein and luteolin. (A) Molecular docking was performed on PatchDock Server. Visualization and bond analysis were done on Chimera: (A) Tertiary structure visualization. (B) Secondary structure. Ligand attached on Chain C (different grey shade) of HPV E6 protein. (B) Docking analysis file read in Protein Ligand Interaction Profiler (PLIP). Interacting chains and the type of bond interactions are tabulated in detail.

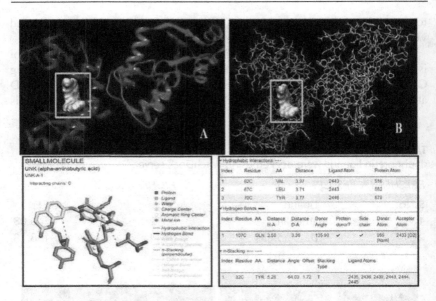

FIGURE 8.9 HPV E6 protein and daphnoretin. (A) Molecular docking was performed on PatchDock Server. Visualization and bond analysis were done on Chimera: (A) Tertiary structure visualization. (B) Secondary structure. Ligand attached on Chain C (different grey shade) of HPV E6 protein. (B) Docking analysis file read in Protein Ligand Interaction Profiler (PLIP). Interacting chains and the type of bond interactions are tabulated in detail.

was done using the Protein Ligand Interaction Profiler (Figures 8.8B and 8.9B). The docking analysis results indicated hydrogen bond and hydrophobic interactions in MD between E6 and luteolin; and hydrogen bonds, hydrophobic interactions, and pie-stacking (perpendicular) interactions in MD between daphnoretin and E6. This analysis strengthens our resolve to continue with these ligands for further studies into a pipeline of ADME analysis.

ADME (absorption, dissolution, metabolism and excretion) properties of both the ligands and the calculated result (physicochemical properties, lipophilicity, water solubility, pharmacokinetics, drug likeliness and medicinal chemistry) are presented in Figure 8.10A and B. Both hits have 0 Lipinski violation, do not pass through the blood-brain barrier (BBB) and have high gastrointestinal absorption. Both ligands further undergo toxicity testing, as presented in Table 8.3.

Further, they were tested for their bioactivity (GPCR ligand, ion channel modulator, kinase inhibitor, nuclear receptor ligand, protease inhibitor and enzyme inhibitor) and for their molecular properties (miLogP, TPSA < natoms, MW, noN, nOHNH, nviolations, nrotb, volume) using Molinspiration.

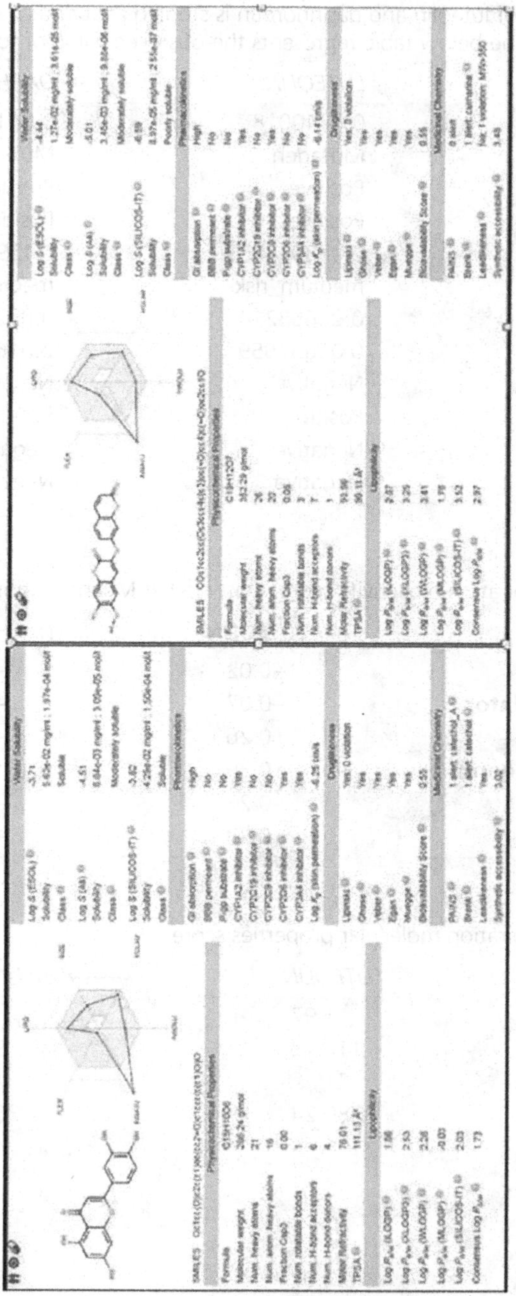

FIGURE 8.10 (A) Different ADME properties of luteolin and (B) daphnoretin.

TABLE 8.3   Toxicity of luteolin and daphnoretin is studied at various parameters on preADMET tool. The below table represents the observed value of toxicity.

PROPERTIES	LUTEOLIN	DAPHNORETIN
Algae_at	0.0340018	0.0416314
Ames_test	Mutagen	Mutagen
Carcino_Mouse	Positive	Positive
Carcino_Rat	Positive	Positive
daphnia_at	0.0580438	0.139325
hERG_inhibition	medium_risk	medium_risk
medaka_at	0.00658214	0.0329883
minnow_at	0.00657559	0.0169052
TA100_10RLI	Negative	Negative
TA100_NA	Positive	Positive
TA1535_10RLI	Negative	Negative
TA1535_NA	Negative	Negative

TABLE 8.4   Molinspiration bioactivity score. Observed at Molinspiration.

PROPERTIES	LUTEOLIN	DAPHNORETIN
GPCR ligand	−0.02	−0.21
Ion channel modulator	−0.07	−0.28
Kinase inhibitor	0.26	−0.13
Nuclear receptor ligand	0.39	0.01
Protease inhibitor	−0.22	−0.21
Enzyme inhibitor	0.28	−0.14

TABLE 8.5   Molinspiration molecular properties score.

PROPERTIES	LUTEOLIN	DAPHNORETIN
MiLogP	1.97	3.06
TPSA	111.12	99.12
Natoms	21	26
MW	286.24	352.30
noN	6	7
nOHNH	4	1
nviolations	0	0
Nrotb	1	3
volume	232.07	287.09

Their scores are tabulated in Tables 8.4 and 8.5. These results tie in well with previously conducted studies wherein similar results were obtained [27–30]. Hence, on the basis of the in silico results, these compounds can serve as potential leads.

FUTURE PROSPECTS AND CLINICAL INTERPRETATION

Drug discovery is an interdisciplinary effort for designing effective and commercially feasible drugs where CADD initiates the process by rationale identification of potential hits which have the ability to develop into successful drugs via clinical trials. Today, treatment for cervical cancer includes immunotherapy, therapeutic vaccines, immune checkpoint inhibitors, chemotherapy, surgery and radiotherapy combinations to attenuate cancerous microenvironment. Recently, electroporation (EP) techniques–based DNA vaccines have demonstrated great potential with increased immunogenicity and efficacy (VGX-3100, which administers HPV 16/18 DNA vaccines by EP is already in phase III clinical trials). Another similar HSP70 DNA vaccine, fused with immuno-stimulatory proteins (NCT00121173) is in phase I and II trials. Other chemical drugs in various stages of clinical trials include AZD5363 or capivasertib (CHEMBL2325741) (NCT01226316) (Phase I); sizofiran (NCT01926821), rucaparib (NCT03795272), HspE7 or verpasep caltespen (NCT00075569), niraparib, dostralimab (NCT04068753) (Phase II); and fenretinide (NCT00003075) (Phase III). However, these methods have adverse side effects. Even with cutting-edge approaches like DNA vaccines, viral DNA administration raises the risk of oncogenicity and obstructs metabolic pathways. Meeting with demands of the time, plant-based drugs and vaccines with lesser side effects and toxicity are in various stages of development. Several herbal drugs including curcumin have been tested in silico and in vitro and have been reported to be active against breast cancer [31]. Based on rational drug designing approaches, Curcumin is currently in phase II testing for radiation-induced dermatitis in breast cancer patients (NCT01042938) and for treatment of advanced metastatic breast cancer (NCT03072992).

As to the proposed two inhibitors of E6 oncoprotein, luteolin is in early Phase I clinical trials for other types of cancer including tongue carcinoma (NCT03288298), and daphnoretin recently patented as an effective treatment against tissue/organ rejection or GVHD [32]. Luteolin is reported to inhibit cell proliferation, survival signalling, angiogenesis and metastasis by inhibiting PI3K-Akt, and it acts on apoptosis by activating DR5 and inhibiting

Bcl-XL in various types of cancers [33]. Daphnoretin is known to exert its anticancer effects through the inhibition of cancer cell proliferation, the induction of G2/M-phase arrest and apoptosis [28]. Synergistic approaches by combining two or more of such herbal-based compounds are also in progress; for example, luteolin with quercetin and rutin are currently being tested for autism spectrum disorder (Phase II) (NCT01847521). Herein we are proposing the use of luteolin and daphnorectin as key inhibitors of HPV E6, and further validation of these in terms of in vitro and preclinical studies are required.

CONCLUSION

In this study, we utilized various computational tools to devise herbal drugs effective against cervical cancer, with lesser side effects and greater effectivity. We targeted the E6 protein with phytochemical ligands (luteolin and daphnoretin), and came to the conclusion that both have the ability to bind to the chain C of E6 protein by several bonds like hydrogen bonds, hydrophobic interactions and pie stacking. Both are predicted to be safe for oral administration as they do not cross the blood-brain barrier and have a higher gastrointestinal absorption rate. They are very likely to pass the further drug tests due to no violation of the Lipinski rule and are safe to use as predicted by the toxicity tests. Taking these results as a basis, lead optimization and chemical modifications can be done. Various phytochemicals can be proposed for clinical trials and treatment of many diseases. Luteolin can offer a comparatively more secure alternative approach for HPV treatment after clinical validations.

SUMMARY

- Recent statistics show that there is a requirement for change regarding current treatment methodologies, together with radiotherapy and chemotherapy.
- The problem of lesser FDA approval (with longer time periods invested) can be combatted by CADD to propose the hits that have major chances of in vitro/in vivo success.
- Here we utilize herbal informatics in combination with CADD to propose luteolin and daphnoretin as potential ligands against HPV (E6 oncoprotein).

- Both the ligands bind to the chain C of the E6 oncoprotein exhibiting hydrophobic interactions, pie stackings and other bonds between the ligands and target molecules by study through interaction profilers.

REFERENCES

1. Basu P, Roychowdhury S, Bafna UD, et al. Human papillomavirus genotype distribution in cervical cancer in India: Results from a multi-center study. *Asian Pac J Cancer Prev.* 2009 January–March;10(1):27–34, PMID: 19469620.
2. Bruni L, Barrionuevo-Rosas L, Albero G, et al. Human papillomavirus and related diseases report. *HPV Information Centre.* 2017;(Summary Report 19 April 2017):60.
3. Crook T, Tidy JA, Vousden KH. Degradation of p53 can be targeted by HPV E6 sequences distinct from those required for p53 binding and trans-activation. *Cell.* 1991 November 1; 67(3):547–556. doi:10.1016/0092-8674(91)90529-8.
4. Leach AR, Harren J. *Structure-Based Drug Discovery.* Berlin: Springer, 2007, doi:10.1021/ja076951v.
5. National center for biotechnology information (NCBI)[Internet]. Bethesda (MD): National library of medicine (US), National center for biotechnology information; [1988]—[cited 2021 September 05], available from www.ncbi.nlm.nih.gov/.
6. The UniProt Consortium. UniProt: The universal protein knowledgebase in 2021. *Nucleic Acids Res.* 2021;49:D1.
7. Gasteiger E, Hoogland C, Gattiker A, et al. Protein identification and analysis tools on the ExPASy server. In John M. Walker (ed): *The Proteomics Protocols Handbook.* Totowa: Humana Press, 2005, 571–607.
8. Geourjon C, Deleage G. SOPMA: Significant improvements in protein secondary structure prediction by consensus prediction from multiple alignments. Institut de Biologie et de Chimie des Proteines, UPR 412-CNRS, Lyon, France. *Comput Appl Biosci.* 1995 December;11(6):681–684.
9. Jones DT. Protein secondary structure prediction based on position-specific scoring matrices. *J. Mol. Biol.* 1999;292: 195–202.
10. Drozdetskiy A, Cole C, Procter J, Barton GJ. (first published online April 16, 2015) JPred4: A protein secondary structure prediction server. *Nucleic Acids Res.* Web Server issue. doi:10.1093/nar/gkv332.
11. Berman HM, Westbrook J, Feng Z, et al. The protein data bank. *Nucleic Acids Res.* 2000;28:235–242.
12. Pettersen EF, Goddard TD, Huang CC, Couch GS, Greenblatt DM, Meng EC, et al. UCSF Chimera-a visualization system for exploratory research and analysis. *J Comput Chem.* 2004 October;25(13):1605–1612.
13. Szklarczyk D, Gable AL, Nastou KC, et al. The STRING database in 2021: Customizable protein—protein networks, and functional characterization of user-uploaded gene/measurement sets. *Nucleic Acids Res.* 2021 January 8;49(D1):D605–612.

14. Kanehisa M, Furumichi M, Sato Y. KEGG: Integrating viruses and cellular organisms. *Nucleic Acids Res.* 2021;49:D545–D551.
15. Majumdar D, Jung KH, Zhang H, et al. Luteolin nanoparticle in chemoprevention: In vitro and in vivo anticancer activity. *Cancer Prev Res (Philadelphia, Pa.).* 2014;7(1):65–73. https://doi.org/10.1158/1940-6207.CAPR-13-0230.
16. National Center for Biotechnology Information. *PubChem Compound Summary for CID 5281406.* Daphnoretin, available September 5, 2021, from https://pubchem.ncbi.nlm.nih.gov/compound/Daphnoretin.
17. Kim S, Chen J, Cheng T, et al. PubChem in 2021: New data content and improved web interfaces. *Nucleic Acids Res.* 2019;49(D1):D1388–D1395. https://doi.org/10.1093/nar/gkaa971.
18. Mendez D, Gaulton A, Bento AP, et al. ChEMBL: Towards direct deposition of bioassay data. *Nucleic Acids Res.* 2019;47(D1):D930–D940. doi:10.1093/nar/gky1075.
19. Wishart DS, Knox C, Guo AC, et al. Drugbank: A comprehensive resource for in silico drug discovery and exploration. *Nucleic Acids Res.* 2006 January 1;34 (Database issue):D668–672.16381955.
20. Schneidman-Duhovny D, Inbar Y, Nussinov R, Wolfson HJ. PatchDock and SymmDock: Servers for rigid and symmetric docking. *Nucl Acids Res.* 2005;33:W363–367.
21. Salentin S., et al. PLIP: Fully automated protein-ligand interaction profiler. *Nucl. Acids Res.* 2015 July 1;43(W1):W443–W447. doi:10.1093/nar/gkv315.
22. Swiss Institute of Bioinformatics. SwissADME: A free web tool to evaluate pharmacokinetics, drug-likeness and medicinal chemistry friendliness of small molecules, available from www.swissadme.ch/.
23. Guan L, Yang H, Cai Y, et al. ADMET-score—a comprehensive scoring function for evaluation of chemical drug-likeness. *MedChemComm.* 2018;10(1):148–157. https://doi.org/10.1039/c8md00472b, available from https://preadmet.bmdrc.kr/.
24. Slovensky G. Slovakia, Molinspiration Cheminformatics free web services, available from www.molinspiration.com.
25. Lin Y, Shi R, Wang X, Shen HM. Luteolin, a flavonoid with potential for cancer prevention and therapy. *Curr Cancer Drug Targets.* 2008;8(7):634–646. https://doi.org/10.2174/156800908786241050.
26. Jiang HF, Wu Z, Bai X, Zhang Y, He P. Effect of daphnoretin on the proliferation and apoptosis of A549 lung cancer cells *in vitro. Oncol Lett.* 2014;8(3):1139–1142. https://doi.org/10.3892/ol.2014.2296.
27. Mamgain S, Sharma P, Pathak RK, Baunthiyal M. Computer aided screening of natural compounds targeting the E6 protein of HPV using molecular docking. *Bioinformation.* 2015;11(5):236–242. https://doi.org/10.6026/97320630011236.
28. Cherry JJ, Rietz A, Malinkevich A, et al. Structure based identification and characterization of flavonoids that disrupt human papillomavirus-16 E6 function. *PloS One.* 2013;8(12):e84506. https://doi.org/10.1371/journal.pone.0084506.
29. Lopez JR, Limon AV, Zunniga M, et al. Molecular modelling simulation studies reveal new potential inhibitors against HPV E6 protein, 2019 March 15. https://doi.org/10.1371/journal.pone.0213028.
30. Ricci-López J, Vidal-Limon A, Zunñiga M, et al. Molecular modeling simulation studies reveal new potential inhibitors against HPV E6 protein. *PloS One.* 2019;14(3):e0213028. https://doi.org/10.1371/journal.pone.0213028.

31. Yim-im W, Sawatdichaikul O, Semsri S, et al. Computational analyses of curcuminoid analogs against kinase domain of HER2. *BMC Bioinformatics.* 2014;15:261. https://doi.org/10.1186/1471-2105-15-261.

32. Chen, et al. Daphnoretin modulates differentiation and maturation of human dendritic cells through down-regulation of c-Jun N-terminal kinase. *Int Immunopharmacol.* 2017 August 1;51:25–30, Elsevier, 2017, PMID: 28772243.

33. Imran M, Rauf A, Abu-Izneid T, et al. Luteolin, a flavonoid, as an anticancer agent: A review. *Biomed Pharmacother.* 2019;112:108612, ISSN 0753–3322, https://doi.org/10.1016/j.biopha.2019.108612.

Advances in Big Data and Machine Learning in Cancer Detection in Women-Associated Cancers

9

Dhaval Kumar Srivastava, Aditya Vikram Singh and Ankur Saxena

Contents

DOI: 10.1201/9781003260172-9

INTRODUCTION

Modern-day technologies like big data and machine learning are being utilized in various stages of cancer research like drug discovery, target validation, biomarker identification, computer-aided processing of images and collection of digital pathology, and this large-scale data is considered for the application of machine learning and big data in cancer diagnostics (Figure 9.2) [1]. Machine learning is a technique for data analysis that carries out analytical model designing. It is a branch of artificial intelligence that is based on the vision that a system can learn from a dataset provided, identifying different patterns in data and make decisions on its own with minimal human interventions. Machine learning can be two types: supervised learning and unsupervised learning, with only one pertaining difference, that is the existence of labels in the datasets (Figure 9.1) [2]. Big data is a field of modern computing that treats ways to analyse, systematically extracts information from, or otherwise deal with data sets that are too large or complex to be dealt with by traditional data-processing application software. Data with many fields (columns) offer greater statistical power, while data with higher complexity (more attributes or columns) may lead to a higher false discovery rate. The amount of data generated from various diagnosis methodologies is significantly large, and this large volume is considered for the application of machine learning and big data in cancer diagnostics. New technologies for big data have emerged and have helped in reducing the cost for storing large amounts of data of women-associated cancers.

STATUS QUO OF MACHINE LEARNING IN WOMEN-ASSOCIATED CANCERS

The investigation of the breast cancer data from the Wisconsin dataset from UCI machine learning to develop accurate prediction models for breast cancer using data mining techniques led to the comparison of three classification techniques utilizing Weka software, wherein the results demonstrated that sequential minimal optimization (SMO) attained a prediction accuracy of 96.2%, higher than that of the LBK and BF Tree methods [3]. Another study has been implemented on medical data from the WDBC directory containing 569 instances and 32 features, where they used feature-selection mechanism to minimize the number of features and utilized K-means clustering algorithm to divide tumours into clusters. Subsequently, the application of hybrid K-SVM model reduced the computational time significantly and obtained a higher accuracy of 97.38% [4]. The impact of gene expression (GE) and DNA methylation (DM) has also been reported, focusing on the study of prediction breast cancer by utilizing genetic data of the patients, where the use of SVM classifier manifested to be potent in breast cancer prediction, as it attained best results in terms of accuracy (96.33%) and precision (97.2%) [5].

A study pertaining to the potential of MALDI-imaging, using linear discriminant analysis (LDA), support vector machines with linear (SVM-lin) and radial basis function kernels (SVM-rbf) for the classification of EOC histological subtypes from tissue microarray and the spectra of 11,749 to 12,059 for the training set, 3,470 for the validation set and 7,361 to 7,512 for the test set, have been evaluated, wherein the classifications of EOC histotypes were obtained with the mean accuracy of 80% for LDA, 80% SVM-lin, and 74% SVM-rbf [6]. An accurate prediction model was proposed for benign ovarian tumours (BOT) and practical value of ovarian cancer (OC) considering a dataset of 349 Chinese patients, utilizing machine learning's minimum redundancy–maximum relevance (MRMR) feature selection, decision tree methods, and the results were compared for the two biomarkers (i.e., HE4 and CEA). The model was simple to interpret and outperformed the existing OC prediction models, but with a limitation of small sample size [7]. Artificial intelligence (AI) and machine learning (ML) have also been sourced to predict the pathological diagnosis of ovarian tumours on the basis of 16 different features by analysing their importance in prediction of the disease, wherein the highest accuracy of 80% in the XG-Boost ML algorithm, followed by 78%, 67%, 62% in random forest, logistic regression, and support vector machine, respectively, have been attained [8]. The use of ML for the prediction of abdominal recurrence of serial cancer antigen 125 (CA125) levels in patients with advanced high-grade serous ovarian cancer based on CT surveillance has also been reported, wherein four measures of CA125 were optimized and evaluated using SVM and tenfold cross-validation to determine the most predictive measure of CA125, and it was found that the rate of change in CA125 was most predictive for abdominal recurrence in a linear kernel SVM model and was significantly higher preceding CT studies showing abdominal recurrence (median 13.2 versus 0.6 units/month; $p = 0.007$) [9].

Multi-parameter magnetic resonance imaging (MRI) and ML have also been utilized to automate the interpretation of colposcopic images, wherein the segmentation of these images based on multiparametric MRI consisting of T2-weighted (T2w), T1-weighted (T1w) and dynamic contrast-enhanced (DCE) sequences has resulted in mean sensitivity of 94% and 52%, respectively, while on including DCE-MR images, the mean sensitivity attained was 93% [10]. Convolutional neural network (CNN) and ML were combined recently to classify cervical cancer using the Herlev database, wherein the proposed system achieved accuracy of 99.5% in the detection problem and of 91.2% in the classification problem [11]. The image analysis techniques have also been reviewed wherein ML approaches were introduced for automatic screening of cervical cancer from Pap smear dataset, which concluded with the efficiency of the KNN and SVM classifiers as 99.27% and 98.5%, respectively [12]. Transfer learning strategies, aiming to extract knowledge from at least one source task and use it when learning a predictive model for a new target task, have also been used for the prediction of the individual patient risk based on a dataset of medical tests from patients with cervical cancer [13].

A prediction model for endometrial cancer (EC) patients has also been constructed using the naïve Bayes ML algorithm for lymph node involvement (LNI) prediction, which reported the necessity of lymphadenectomy and the prediction of LNI in endometrial cancer, wherein it assessed 762 patients with EC based on the histopathological factors and in the mean age of patients of 59.1 years, LNI was detected in 102 (13.4%) patients, and para-aortic LNI (PaLNI) was detected in 54 (7.1%) patients. The accuracy rate of the algorithm models for LNI and PaLNI was found to be between 84.2% and 88.9% and 85.0% and 97.6%, respectively [14]. In a recent study, the identification of deep myometrial invasion (DMI) in endometrial cancer (EC) patients, and its clinical applicability has been investigated using an MRI radiomics-powered ML model, wherein out of the extracted 1,132 features after feature selection, the classifier reached an accuracy of 86% and 91%. The areas under the receiver operating characteristic curve of cross-validation and final testing gave accuracies of 92% and 94%, respectively [15].

STATUS QUO OF BIG DATA IN WOMEN-ASSOCIATED CANCERS

Although big data is a separate field, most of its work is based upon machine learning methodologies.

Radiotherapy of tumours in breast cancer requires accurate, patient-specific treatment, and in general, such segmentation is performed by manual delineation using computed tomography (CT) and/or magnetic resonance (MR) imaging techniques. However, manual delineation is challenging and time-consuming and hence, accurate automated segmentation methods are highly desired for pre-treatment and adaptive radiotherapy planning during treatments [16]. Zhang et al. trained a very deep dilated residual network (DD-ResNet) for fast and consistent auto-segmentation performance of the proposed model, which was then evaluated against two different deep learning models: the deep dilated convolutional neural network (DDCNN) and the deep deconvolutional neural network (DDNN). The mean dice similarity coefficient (DSC) values attained for DD-ResNet (0.91 and 0.91) were higher than the other two networks (DDCNN: 0.85; mean segmentation time was 4 s, 21 s and 15 s per patient with DDCNN, DDNN and DD-ResNet, respectively) [16].

Yashoda and Anathanarayanan incorporated feature selection and classification to develop a predictive model for ovarian cancer detection. A large amount of data was gathered to build knowledge-based system and a rough set theory, which was then utilized to find the data reliance. The hybrid particle genetic swarm optimization (PGSO) was used to optimize the selected features for efficient classification for different stages of ovarian cancer, followed by multiclass SVM, which was adopted as the classifier to classify normal or different stages of ovarian cancer using the optimized feature set, the proposed system when compared with the ANN and naïve Bayes achieved 96% accuracy for dataset I and 98% accuracy for dataset II [17].

Zhang and Cheng have studied the application of big data in early diagnosis and the treatment of human papillomavirus (HPV)–infected cervical cancer patients. They utilized a traditional ID3-based decision tree model, which was then optimized through the minimum sample number of different leaf nodes, and the diagnosis model for cervical cancer patients was constructed. Diagnosis model and information monitoring system (DMIMS) was compared with the decision tree based on decision support degree (DTBDS), to this, results depicted that the classification accuracy of DMIMS (95%) was higher than that of DTBDS (67%), suggesting that the big data monitoring system of cervical cancer plays an important role in the detection of HPV-infection cervical cancer [18].

The rate of inguinal lymph node metastasis is relatively low in cervical cancer patients, and according to the National Comprehensive Cancer Network (NCCN) guidelines for cervical cancer, patients with stages invading the lower third of the vagina require bilateral inguinal lymphatic area preventive irradiation [19]. Wang et al. reported the study of the requirement of preventive inguinal area irradiation, wherein they selected a total of 184 patients with cervical cancer accompanied with the lower third of vaginal invasion, and conducted a trial and control method for selecting 180 patients without inguinal lymph node metastasis; 13 cases (7.07%) of 184 patients were found with inguinal lymph node enlargement by imaging examination, and only four cases (2.17%) were further confirmed by pathology. They concluded that even if they do not perform preventive inguinal lymph node irradiation, there is no difference in the recurrence rate of inguinal lymph nodes. They also found that the vaginal wall of two patients with inguinal lymph node metastasis was deeply invaded and reached the vaginal opening; to this, they concluded that preventive radiotherapy might be required for those patients with deep vaginal wall invasion, which requires big data analysis of multiple centres and more cases [19].

CONCLUSION

New big data and machine learning technologies have evolved, lowering the cost of maintaining massive amounts of data related to women's malignancies. The necessity for observable symptoms that a general practitioner (GP) can recognize as an augury of a cancer diagnosis is a major limiting factor in early cancer detection. However, it is possible to identify mutagens that increase the risk for a given cancer type and determine new biomarkers for detection by collecting data on whether the cancer is detected clinically or through screening, the stage of diagnosis, data on exposures and lifestyle, and data from the cellular and molecular levels (through the power of genome-wide surveys). By combining the power of AI with these enormous datasets, new possibilities have emerged. The need of classifying cancer patients into high- or low-risk categories has prompted numerous research teams in the biomedical and bioinformatics fields to investigate the use of machine learning (ML) algorithms for modelling cancer development and treatment. The majority of current research has focused on the construction of predictive models employing supervised machine learning approaches and classification of algorithms in order to anticipate valid treatment methodologies (Figure 9.1). Based on their findings, it is clear that the integration of multidimensional heterogeneous data, together with the use of various approaches such as feature selection and classification, might give promising inference tools in the cancer sphere. Even while it is clear that the application of machine learning algorithms can help us better understand cancer progression, these technologies need to be validated before they can be used in clinical practice (Figure 9.2).

REFERENCES

1. Dlamini Z, Francies FZ, Hull R, Marima R. Artificial intelligence (AI) and big data in cancer and precision oncology. *Computational and Structural Biotechnology Journal.* 2020;18:2300–2311.
2. Gupta M, Srivastava DK, Sreedharan SM, et al. Investigating the Impact of COVID-19 Crisis on The Economy of USA and India: A Comparative Study Using Machine Learning. *Turkish Journal of Physiotherapy and Rehabilitation.* 2021;32(2):3739–3799.

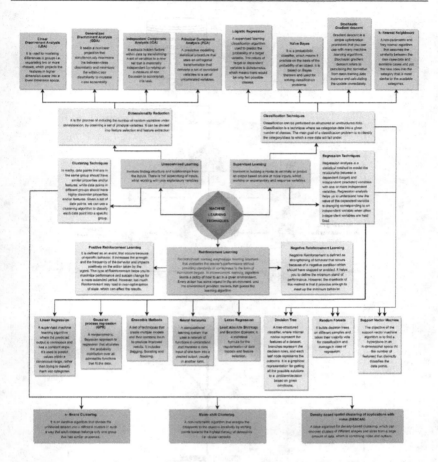

FIGURE 9.1 Classification of ML algorithms. Systematics classification of ML algorithms, which incorporate supervised, unsupervised and reinforced learning and their further classification.

3. Chaurasia V, Pal S. A Novel Approach for Breast Cancer Detection Using Data Mining Techniques. *International Journal of Innovative Research in Computer and Communication Engineering* (An ISO 3297: 2007 Certified Organization). 2014 January;2(1).

4. Zheng B, Yoon SW, Lam SS. Breast cancer diagnosis based on feature extraction using a hybrid of K-means and support vector machine algorithms. *Expert Systems with Applications*. 2014 Mar;41(4):1476–1482.

5. Alghunaim S, Al-Baity HH. On the Scalability of Machine-Learning Algorithms for Breast Cancer Prediction in Big Data Context. *IEEE Access*. 2019;7:91535–91546.

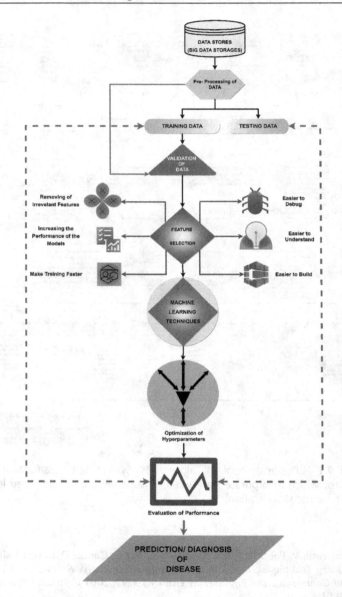

FIGURE 9.2 Machine learning workflow. A typical machine learning pipeline starts from attaining the dataset and ends when the desired results are obtained. The internal environment incorporates steps including pre-processing, dataset distribution, validation, feature-selection, application of ML algorithms, optimization of hyperparameters, and evaluation of performance, wherein these steps keep repeating themselves until the desired results are obtained.

6. Klein O, Kanter F, Kulbe H, Jank P, Denkert C, Nebrich G, et al. MALDI-Imaging for Classification of Epithelial Ovarian Cancer Histotypes from a Tissue Microarray Using Machine Learning Methods. *Proteomics Clinical Applications.* 2019 Jan;13(1):1700181.

7. Lu M, Fan Z, Xu B, Chen L, Zheng X, Li J, et al. Using machine learning to predict ovarian cancer. *International Journal of Medical Informatics.* 2020 Sept;141:104195.

8. Akazawa M, Hashimoto K. Artificial Intelligence in Ovarian Cancer Diagnosis. *Anticancer Research.* 2020 Aug;40(8):4795–800.

9. Shinagare AB, Balthazar P, Ip IK, Lacson R, Liu J, Ramaiya N, et al. High-Grade Serous Ovarian Cancer: Use of Machine Learning to Predict Abdominopelvic Recurrence on CT on the Basis of Serial Cancer Antigen 125 Levels. *Journal of the American College of Radiology.* 2018 Aug;15(8):1133–1138.

10. Torheim T, Malinen E, Hole KH, Lund KV, Indahl UG, Lyng H, et al. Auto delineation of cervical cancers using multiparametric magnetic resonance imaging and machine learning. *Acta Oncologica.* 2017 May 4;56(6):806–812.

11. Ghoneim A, Muhammad G, Hossain MS. Cervical cancer classification using convolutional neural networks and extreme learning machines. *Future Generation Computer Systems.* 2020 Jan;102:643–649.

12. William W, Ware A, Basaza-Ejiri AH, Obungoloch J. A review of image analysis and machine learning techniques for automated cervical cancer screening from pap-smear images. *Computer Methods and Programs in Biomedicine.* 2018 Oct;164:15–22.

13. Fernandes K, Cardoso JS, Fernandes J. Transfer Learning with Partial Observability Applied to Cervical Cancer Screening. In: Alexandre L., Salvador Sánchez J., Rodrigues J. (eds) Pattern Recognition and Image Analysis. IbPRIA 2017. *Lecture Notes in Computer Science*, 2017, vol. 10255. Springer, Cham. https://doi.org/10.1007/978-3-319-58838-4_27.

14. Günakan E, Atan S, Haberal AN, et al. A novel prediction method for lymph node involvement in endometrial cancer: machine learning. *International Journal of Gynecologic Cancer* 2019;29:320–324.

15. Stanzione A, Cuocolo R, Del Grosso R, Nardiello A, Romeo V, Travaglino A, et al. Deep Myometrial Infiltration of Endometrial Cancer on MRI: A Radiomics-Powered Machine Learning Pilot Study. *Academic Radiology.* 2021 May;28(5):737–744.

16. Men K, Zhang T, Chen X, Chen B, Tang Y, Wang S, et al. Fully automatic and robust segmentation of the clinical target volume for radiotherapy of breast cancer using big data and deep learning. *Physica Medica.* 2018 Jun;50:13–19.

17. Yasodha P, Ananthanarayanan NR. Analysing Big Data to Build Knowledge Based System for Early Detection of Ovarian Cancer. *Indian Journal of Science and Technology.* 2015 Jul 9;8(14).

18. Chen G, Zhang W. Application of big data information system in early diagnosis, treatment, and nursing of cervical cancer infected by human papillomavirus. *Expert Systems.* 2021;31.

19. Wang L, Huang K, Wang Y, et al. Discussion on the Necessity of Bilateral Inguinal Lymphatic Area Irradiation for Cervical Cancer with Invasion of the Lower One Third of Vagina. *Research Square*, 2020;8.

Clinicians' Perspective in the Use and Adaptability of the Latest Methods of Diagnosis and Treatment for Cancers in Women

10

Umme Abiha and Charu Sharma

DOI: 10.1201/9781003260172-10

Contents

INTRODUCTION

The primitive era of pathology is evolving at a rapid pace. The transformation into the digital management of tissue samples, reports and histopathological diagnosis has been achieved through integrated platforms of artificial intelligence (AI) and machine learning (ML). It has successively proceeded towards cost- and time-efficient diagnostic tools which aid in the early prognosis of diseases [1]. Moreover, the evolution of whole-slide imaging scanners which abandon the primitive use of optical microscopes is similar to radiological imaging; however, the extent of analogy remains a concern due to the dense barrier in histology. At the same time, it is even difficult to establish a complete analogy due to the difference in availability of primary object of analysis. This has even seen its application in other diverse fields of diseases, and cancer is one of the popular research subjects.

Today, the most prevalent types of carcinomas (cervical cancer and breast cancer) are being extensively studied and analysed using the approach of image analysis [2]. The need of improvement in tedious procedures of analysis of the histological grade and hormone receptor status of breast cancer by immunohistochemistry (IHC) was a potential reason behind fuelling the research in this direction.

DIAGNOSING BREAST CANCER USING IMAGE ANALYSIS

The area of research focusing on the analysis of breast cancer histopathological images has gained much traction in the scientific community. One of the biggest drivers was the need that was unanimously felt in the pathological workflow at all places. This has transformed according to the current need for analysis. The tedious work and long waiting hours depending on the observer's variability that often leads to a suspicion of doubt came with an instant solution of whole-slide imaging (WSI) scanners. This economical and automatic high-throughput slide digitization scanned the images at 20× or 40× magnification with a spatial resolution on the order of 0.50 µm/pixel and 0.25 µm/pixel, respectively. The captured RGB image is compressed in JPEG or JPEG 2000 and then stored in a pyramid structure with increasing magnification at each level [3].

This further facilitates multiscale image analysis. However, this comes with a few precautions while performing tissue preparation, staining and slide digitization processes which carries a significant impact on analysis using image analysis algorithms.

The hormone receptor status in breast cancer is the crucial step in planning any adjuvant systemic treatment, which begins with scoring immunohistochemistry (IHC)-stained slides via visual examination under a microscope. Recently, the American Society of Clinical Oncology and the College of American Pathologists for testing of the estrogen receptors (ER), progesterone receptors (PR), and human epidermal growth factor receptor-2 (HER2) receptor status focused on the use of quantitative image analysis techniques to reduce the variability in interpretation [4–5]. Furthermore, the hormone receptor status is determined by counting the percentage number of positively stained nuclei while the automatic image analysis system that quantifies ER and PR status upon the use of an automated nuclei detection and segmentation algorithm [6]. Comparing these two, HER2 is expressed on the cell membrane, and this tumour is taken positive only when >10% of the cell membrane is positively stained [4].

The images of the stained region are pixels that are classified as either belonging to epithelial nuclei or cell membranes, whereas the nuclear regions are segmented into individual nuclei by watershed segmentation and the cell membranes are determined by adaptive ellipse fitting. These are then classified into one of the three scoring groups based on features describing the membrane staining intensity and completeness. Numerous other studies have been reported showing automatic scoring using fluorescent in situ hybridization (FISH) for HER2 scoring [7–8].

Despite efforts in solving the challenges of nuclei segmentation in breast histopathology images, it remains a concern. This is due to differences in tissue appearance, diversity in epithelial cancerous nuclei, and overlapping of nuclei and hematoxylin-stained junk particles which appear in high-grade tumours. All these hamper the nuclei segmentation. With the noted hindrances that occur in routine pathological practice, the biggest obstacle is the unavailability of large annotated datasets. Although the advent of WSI scanners has produced enormous quantities of image data, it is still difficult to obtain ground truth annotations in a form that can be used readily for developing and testing image analysis methods.

PERSPECTIVES ON EARLY DETECTION AND SCREENING OF CERVICAL CANCER

Cervical cancer is a serious concern to a women's health, with incident cases of 604,127 and mortality rate of 341,831 individuals worldwide [9]. The control of this disease comes with the intervention of screening, meaning the early detection of precancerous changes in women. Various screening programmes are being encouraged at the central level to check for the high prevalence of human papillomavirus (HPV) infection and incidence of cervical precancer and invasive cancer. Since this is one cancer which has a long latent period and the fact that "precancerous lesions are curable," there is a huge responsibility on the clinicians to timely diagnose cervical cancer in its precancerous stage by the available screening methods.

Screening of Cervical Cancer

There are four existing modalities for screening cervical cancer:

1. *Cytology screening*: This includes the Papanicolaou (Pap) test, where cells are extracted from the transition zone (T-zone) of the cervix with the help of a spatula or a brush. The collected cells are

then smeared onto a glass slide, stained with Papanicolaou stain and examined under the microscope to determine the abnormality of cells and later classified using Bethesda classification.

Liquid-based cytology (LBC) is another test that is more expensive than a Pap test, where the sample is transferred from a brush to a preservative solution to create a suspension of cells that is later fixed onto a slide. Although expensive, it is preferred as it decreases the number of unsatisfactory smears by eliminating inflammatory cells and red blood cells from background, forms a monolayer smear and has the advantage of reduced reporting time and simultaneous HPV testing.

2. *Visual inspection*: VIA (visual inspection with acetic acid) and VILI (visual inspection with Lugol's iodine) are promising alternatives to cytology, having an average sensitivity of 86% in detecting abnormal lesions. An experimental study validates the effective sensitivity of Lugol's iodine test up to 100% in detection of lesions [10]. The clinicians can effectively treat women with the positive visual inspection tests through cryotherapy. This approach (screen and treat) involves one or two visits with a few follow-ups to track and treat the disease at an early stage.

3. *HPV testing*: The diagnosis of high-risk HPV infection in the cervix requires an expensive and sophisticated laboratory equipment and setup. Currently, it is achieved through detection of HPV in vaginal and cervical smears by hybrid capture 2 assay. It is impossible to completely introduce the whole testing program for HPV in developing countries, as it requires more laboratory facilities and is expensive in comparison to Pap tests.

4. *Colposcopy*: Considered as a sort of secondary screening method in which the lesions are visualized in a magnified view through a green or blue filter. The suspicious area on colposcopy can be biopsied or treated according to the type of lesion.

Diagnosing Cervical Cancer Using Image Analysis

Automated diagnosis and classification of cervical lesions from Pap smear images is in high demand in the current scenario. This technique of whole-slide image scan is able to detect high-grade squamous intraepithelial lesions (HSILs) or frank squamous cell carcinomas (SCCs). The conventional manual analysis of Pap smear images as well as cervical biopsy images is a labour-intensive, time-consuming and error-prone job with a high chance of inter-observer variation. With the advancements in computer technology and artificial intelligence, deep learning or machine learning is being adopted in the diagnosis and classification of cervical lesions. This will help the clinicians to have timely and accurate reports [11–12].

CURRENT AVAILABILITY OF DIAGNOSTIC AND THERAPEUTIC OPTIONS IN CERVICAL AND BREAST CANCERS

The validation on diagnosis of a carcinoma comes with a punch biopsy from the edge of a tumour. Evidences of scientific research and experiments validate the prevalence of squamous cell carcinoma up to 90%, followed by 10% adenocarcinoma and 1% mesonephric carcinoma. The diagnosis is accompanied by formulating the effective therapy for an individual patient. This comes with deriving a correlation of the staging of disease to the patient prognosis. The International Federation of Gynecology and Obstetrics (FIGO) provides a classification of stages based on tumour size and the extent of the disease in the pelvis and other distant organs [13].

Figures 10.1 and 10.2 show the existing modalities of screening, diagnosing and treatments of breast cancer and cervical cancer, respectively.

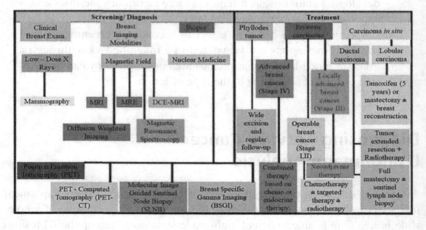

FIGURE 10.1 Modalities for screening, diagnosis and treatment of breast cancer [14].

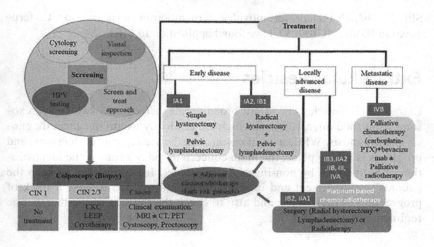

FIGURE 10.2 Modalities for screening, diagnosis and treatment of cervical cancer.

DEMYSTIFYING NEW TREATMENT OPTIONS IN CERVICAL CANCER AND BREAST CANCER

The heterogeneous nature of cancer cells can be studied at both spatial and temporal levels to administer treatment options. There are documented evidences of scientific research that suggests the beginning of new developments of cancer diagnostics and therapeutics [15].

Nanoparticles

Nanoparticles with peculiar properties have offered the abandonment of conventional treatments by providing advantages of high biocompatibility and bioavailability of nanodrugs. The additional advantage of engineering nanoparticles for precision therapy has led research into immunotherapy and the action of drugs to specific stimulus. Quantum dots and superparamagnetic iron oxide (SPIONs) are a few examples of the contrast agents that are used in diagnosis of cancers. Quantum dots due to high fluorescence have proved to be an alternative to photobleaching for imaging and detection purpose, while

SPIONs, which include ferumoxides, ferucarbotran, ferucarbotran C, ferumoxtran 10 and NC100150, have found application in MRI.

Extracellular Vesicles

Extracellular vesicles (EVs) are broadly categorized into two types, exosomes and shed microvesicles, which are clinically useful in cancer diagnosis and prognosis. While a lot of research in the area of cancer diagnosis and prognosis is taking place, the main concern in today's time is the identification of biomarkers by non-invasive techniques. It is important to keep the patients' pre-treatment and intra-treatment information to have a track of progression of the disease and also to check the efficacy of the therapeutic regimen.

Natural Antioxidants

Natural antioxidants including vitamins, polyphenols and plant-derived bioactive compounds in response to the oxidative stress and radical oxygen species act by preventing the damage of DNA and other biomacromolecules in metabolic pathways. Curcumin, a polyphenolic compound extracted from turmeric has anti-inflammatory, antioxidant and chemopreventive properties in brain, lungs and pancreatic cancer. Quercetin and berberine are polyphenolic flavonoid and alkaloid compounds, respectively, that are studied extensively for their chemopreventive and cytotoxic properties.

Targeted Therapy

The disadvantage of conventional therapies is the low specificity of the drugs, and hence a lot of effort is being put in finding a way towards targeted sites. Various receptors and small peptides or proteins are studied for active targeting.

1. The tumour cells have overexpressed receptors, mainly for biotin and folic acid, whose nanocarriers have been designed to target ovarian and endometrial cancers.
2. The others are antibodies which are also equally exploited for such studies. Rapamycin-PLGA nanoparticles conjugated to antibodies exhibit high cellular uptake by human breast adenocarcinoma cells (MCF7) with enhanced apoptotic activity. A number of antibodies have been tested and approved by the FDA for immunotherapy,

including rituximab, ibritumomab tiuxetan, trastuzumab emtansine, nivolumab and pembrolizumab.

3. Anti-angiogenic agents: Gynecology Oncology Group (GOG) 240 is a phase III randomized controlled trial to study the effect of adding bevacizumab to systemic chemotherapy in recurrent, persistent or metastatic cervical cancers [16].

4. Poly-adenosine diphosphate ribose polymerase (PARP) inhibitors: BRCA1 and BRCA2 genes are essential for maintaining genomic stability by ensuring an error free repair of DNA double-stranded breaks through the homologous recombination (HR) repair pathway. Patients with BRCA1 and BRCA2 mutations have tumour cells which are HR deficient, and hence need an alternative pathway which is modulated by PARP. The three common PARP inhibitors approved by FDA are olaparib, rucaparib and niraparib, and are currently in use for ovarian cancers. Research and development in this direction has yielded fruitful results and is bringing us closer to management of cervical cancer [17].

5. Tyrosine kinase inhibitors (TKIs) such as cediranib, nintedanib, sunitinib and pazopanib have also been approved for ovarian cancers and are being studied for cervical cancers.

Radiotherapy and Chemotherapy

Radiotherapy is another popular treatment that is used for women with inoperable cervical cancer or higher-stage cancers with or without chemotherapy. For stage IB3 and IIA2 cervical cancer, primary concurrent chemoradiation (CCRT) is the standard of care, whereas platinum-based chemotherapy (carboplatin and paclitaxel combination) is given for palliative care to reduce the symptoms of distant metastatic cervical cancer.

Gene Therapy

Gene therapy dates back to 1990, when a retroviral vector was exploited to deliver the adenosine deaminase (ADA) gene to T cells in patients with severe combined immunodeficiency (SCID). Over the years, this treatment has evolved in respect to all major cancers to minimize the off-target side effects and increase the effectiveness to specific genes. Folate receptor is a membrane-bound protein which mediates folate uptake by endocytosis, essential for DNA synthesis, cell division and growth, which adds an advantage during malignancy. This was targeted with the development of the folate receptor targeting nano-liposomes to deliver a pigment epithelium-derived factor (PEDF) gene to HeLa cells showing high transfection efficiency and effective anti-tumour activity. This forms the basis that there are multiple ways to target malignancy, especially based on molecules that express themselves on their surface [15].

Thermal Ablation and Cryotherapy

Thermal ablation and magnetic hyperthermia are currently used in treating neoplastic tissues. Thermal ablation uses a temperature lower than $-40°C$ or higher than $60°C$ for long exposure to damage a tumour cell. Hypothermic ablation occurs due to the formation of ice crystals upon cooling, which destroys cell membranes and kills cells. Radiofrequency ablation (RF ablation) is the most popular in clinics because of its efficacy and safety. It uses an alternative current of RF waves to a target zone by an insulated electrode tip and the interaction of the current causes the oscillation of ions in the extracellular fluid which produces heat. Ablation of the T-zone with cryotherapy has been highly successful in curing cervical cancers, as has been reported in a recent Cochrane systematic review, which reports the rate of success in cryotherapy to treat CIN 3 lesions up to 93% [18]. Magnetic hyperthermia is another new way to heat tumour tissues which exploits superparamagnetic or ferromagnetic nanoparticles capable of generating heat after stimulation with an alternating magnetic field [19].

STRENGTHS AND LIMITATIONS OF ADVANCED TREATMENT OPTIONS

Table 10.1 contains a brief overview of strengths and shortcomings of various cancer treatment strategies.

TABLE 10.1 Strengths and shortcomings of innovative cancer treatment strategies.

TREATMENT STRATEGIES	ADVANTAGES	DISADVANTAGES
Nanoparticles	• Highly stable and specific. • High biocompatibility and bioavailability.	• Dependent on the specific nanoparticle.

TREATMENT STRATEGIES	ADVANTAGES	DISADVANTAGES
Extracellular vesicles (EVs)	• Molecular characterization. • High biocompatibility. • In vitro modifiable.	• Lack of preclinical procedures for isolation, quantification, storage and drug loading.
Natural antioxidants	• Easy availability in large quantity. • Exploitation of intrinsic properties.	• Finite bioavailability. • Possible toxicity.
Targeted therapy	• Highly specific. • Reduction of adverse reactions.	• Lack of information regarding long-term side effects.
Gene therapy	• Expression of pro-apoptotic and chemo-sensitizing genes. • Expression of wild-type tumour suppressor genes. • Expression of genes towards specific anti-tumour immune responses. • Targeted silencing of oncogenes and safety by RNA-Interference (RNAi).	• Genome integration. • Limited efficacy in specific subsets of patients. • Higher chances of neutralization by immune system. • Off-target effects and inflammation (RNAi). • Need of delivery systems (RNAi). • Set-up of doses and suitable conditions for controlled release (RNAi).
Thermal ablation	• Treatment is location specific. • Possibility of treatment with MRI imaging.	• Higher efficacy for localized areas. • Low penetration power. • Need for a skilled operator for treatment.
Radiomics/pathomics	• Creation of tumour whole tridimensional volume by non-invasive imaging techniques. Therapeutic and prognostic indicators of disease outcome.	• Need for standardization of procedures to facilitate clinical translation. Description of parameters/ computational/statistical methods to set robust protocols for the generation of models for therapy.

CONCLUSION

To conclude, these advanced image-based analysis methods, being less labour-intensive and less time-consuming, will help clinicians to timely treat the lesions in their precancerous forms and will be a boon in reducing the global burden of female cancers.

SUMMARY

- The International Federation of Gynecology and Obstetrics (FIGO) provides a classification of stages based on tumour size and the extent of the disease in the pelvis and other distant organs.
- The advent of WSI scanners has produced enormous quantities of image data, but it is still difficult to obtain ground truth annotations in a form that can be used readily for developing and testing image analysis methods.
- Image analysis is a revolutionizing field in the area of rapid diagnosis of cervical cancer.
- The new treatment options for cervical and breast cancers have navigated research in new dimensions, fuelling the development of integrated technologies based on artificial intelligence and machine learning.

REFERENCES

1. Harrer S, Shah P, Antony B, *et al.*, Trends Pharmacol Sci (2019). PMID: 31326235 / DOI: 10.1016/j.tips.2019.05.005.
2. Debelee TG, Kebede SR, Schwenker F, *et al.*, J Imaging (2020). PMID: 34460565 / DOI: 10.3390/jimaging6110121.
3. Veta M, Pluim JPW, Van Diest PJ, *et al.*, IEEE Trans Biomed Eng (2014). PMID: 24759275 / DOI: 10.1109/TBME.2014.2303852.
4. Wolff AC, Hammond MEH, Allison KH, *et al.*, Arch Pathol Lab Med (2018). PMID: 29846104 / DOI: 10.5858/arpa.2018-0902-SA.
5. Allison KH, Hammond MEH, Dowsett M, *et al.*, Arch Pathol Lab Med (2020). PMID: 29846104 / DOI: 10.5858/arpa.2018–0902-SA

6. Shamai G, Binenbaum Y, Slossberg R, *et al.*, JAMA Netw Open (2019). PMID: 31348505 / DOI: 10.1001/jamanetworkopen.2019.7700
7. Press MF, Sauter G, Buyse M, *et al.*, J Clin Oncol (2016). PMID: 27573653 / DOI: 10.1200/JCO.2016.66.6693
8. Van der Logt EMJ, Kuperus DAJ, Van Setten JW, *et al.*, PloS One (2015). PMID: 25844540 / DOI: 10.1371/journal.pone.0123201
9. GLOBOCAN 2020: New Global Cancer Data. Available from: www.uicc.org/news/globocan-2020-new-global-cancer-data. [cited 2021 Oct 17].
10. Ghosh P, Gandhi G, Kochhar PK, *et al.*, Indian J Med Res. (2012). PMID: 22960894 / PMCID: PMC3461739
11. Wang C-W, Liou Y-A, Lin Y-J, *et al.*, Sci Rep. (2021). PMID: 34376717 / DOI: 10.1038/s41598-021-95545-y
12. Holmström O, Linder N, Kaingu H, *et al.*, JAMA Netw Open. (2021). PMID: 33729503 / DOI: 10.1001/jamanetworkopen.2021.1740
13. Bhatla N, Berek JS, Cuello Fredes M, *et al.*, Int J Gynaecol Obste. (2019). PMID: 30656645 / DOI: 10.1002/ijgo.12749
14. Zhang B-N, Cao X-C, Chen J-Y, *et al.*, Gland Surg. (2012). PMID: 25083426 / DOI: 10.3978/j.issn.2227-684X.2012.04.07
15. Áyen Á, Jiménez Martínez Y, Boulaiz H. Targeted Gene Delivery Therapies for Cervical Cancer. Cancers (Basel). (2020). PMID: 32455616 / DOI: 10.3390/cancers12051301
16. Tewari KS, Sill MW, Penson RT, *et al.*, Lancet Lond Engl. (2017). PMID: 28756902 / DOI: 10.1016/S0140-6736(17)31607-0
17. Bianchi A, Lopez S, Altwerger G, *et al.*, Gynecol Oncol. (2019). PMID: 31434613 / DOI: 10.1016/j.ygyno.2019.08.010
18. Martin-Hirsch PP, Paraskevaidis E, Bryant A, *et al.* Cochrane Database Syst Rev (2010). PMID: 31434613 / DOI: 10.1016/j.ygyno.2019.08.010
19. Liger_CureMedical-Thermocoagulator-Case-Study-World (2019). Available from: https://viaglobalhealth.com/wp-content/uploads/2020/06/Liger_CureMedical-Thermocoagulator-Case-Study-World-2019.pdf [cited 2021 Oct 17].

Index

Note: *Italicized* page numbers in this index refer to illustrative material.

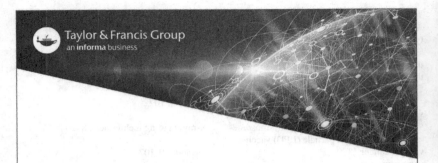

Printed in the United States
by Baker & Taylor Publisher Services

Printed in the United States
by Baker & Taylor Publisher Services